"It is very rare that such a commonsensical and user friendly description of back pain and everyday modalities of treatment and conservative approaches can be so easily elucidated... Certainly I would recommend it to all of my patients."

–Thomas P. Ragukonis, M.D.
Clinical Assistant Professor, Dept. of Anesthesiology
Rutgers New Jersey Medical School (UMDNJ)
Diplomat American Board of Anesthesiology
Diplomat American Board of Pain Medicine

"Dr. Gigante has been one of the great perks of my medical career and he has helped make it so rewarding. By the way, the book is pretty good too!"

–Jerald B. Hershman, MD
Internal Medicine

"Dr. Gigante would have excelled in any profession he chose, luckily for his patients and my profession, he chose chiropractic."

–Gregory P. LaGana, DC
Chiropractic Physician

"This is a 'must read' book for the health professional as well as for the lay person to develop a clear understanding of dealing with a back injury."

–Sammy Masri, MD
Sports Medicine

DR. ALFRED GIGANTE

Chiropractic Physician and Founder of The Back Pain Center

HOPE & HELP

FOR

BACK

PAIN

HOPE AND HELP FOR BACK PAIN
ISBN: 978-0-9970621-5-1
Author: Alfred Gigante, D.C.

3rd Printing, June 2020
2nd Printing, August 2016
1st Printing, January 2016
Printed in the United States of America

First and foremost, I want to thank God for the many blessings in my life.

To my wife, Jeannie, my greatest blessing; thank you for your encouragement, understanding, and love. Your wisdom and sympathetic heart have helped guide us through the highs and lows of life and I am grateful to continue on this journey with you.

To my four children: Alfred, Michael, Daniel, and Jeanmarie, all of whom I love very much. Thank you for adding so much depth and spice to our lives. To my grandchildren Alfred and John and the 2 on the way. *Pure Joy!!*

I'm thankful for my parents; especially for the constants of my mom's love and patience. In 1949, at the age of 29, my mother moved to America from Naples, Italy, leaving behind a life of devastation. Refusing to let her past embitter her family's future, my mom chose a life of compassion, forgiveness, and unconditional love. For this, I am eternally grateful.

To my brothers Jerry & Joey, I'm thankful our bond has not faded in time. To Annmarie, my "baby sister," who has given so unselfishly to our mom. Jerry, Joey and I can never thank you enough.

Thank you Joanne Bonwick, who, after 35 years of keeping order in a whirlwind of changes and new ideas, decided to pass the baton to Melanie. And a big thank you to Melanie who grabbed that baton and didn't miss a step.

To Eric, Steve, Travis, Chetali, Kristel, Cassidy & Lucinda, thank you for your friendship and your loyalty to this office, and most important, your dedication to our patients.

To Gregory LaGana, my "one and only friend" and Columbia Chiropractic classmate, who passed away in April of 2019. I miss you driving me crazy with your never ending Bob Dylan quotes.

Lastly, thank you to my patients for trusting me with your care. Your stories of how Chiropractic has positively impacted your life mean the world to me and the practice. Thank you for your perspective and commitment, which drives me to be better each day.

Table of Contents

Chapter 1
Back Pain

The New Epidemic

It can be said that our greatest quest in life is to pursue that which brings us the greatest joy and meaning. We pursue it in different ways, creating specific goals that we believe will bring us closer to living fully. Most often it includes being active and engaging with friends and family in a wide range of pleasant and productive activities. We love to *feel* great – physically and emotionally – and we embrace many things to help us achieve it.

Yet, other circumstances can hinder our ability to do so. This book focuses on one of those primary obstacles: Back Pain.

This is not earth-shattering news. Undoubtedly, back pain has always afflicted men and women throughout history – but it is getting worse. In fact, back pain is one of the most prevalent medical conditions facing people in this country today. Yet, ironically, it is seldom mentioned when the media highlights some new emerging "epidemic," such as the recent increasing waves of obesity, diabetes, or eating disorders.

Consider this startling fact: approximately 85% of the entire population of the United States will experience back pain at some time in their lives. How many other medical conditions can claim to be so widespread?

It may not always be chronic or long lasting, though for many it can be. The fact that you are reading this book may hint that it's something affecting your life right now. It may be something new to you, or something you've been dealing with on and off for a long time. It may be a source of recurring frustration for you, especially if you've tried different "remedies" and found them to be of limited value. You may feel like nobody can understand what you are going through.

You Are Not Alone

Sometimes when in pain, we think few others can sympathize. We may even be embarrassed by our condition and choose to hide our discomfort from friends or employers, fearing that they are getting tired of our complaints. But, believe me when I say that this problem is far more widespread than most people realize.

Beyond the shocking statistic that 85 percent of the U.S. population will at some point have back pain, let me offer some additional numbers that provide a deeper understanding of the situation:

> ➤ 93 million workdays are lost each year due to back pain
> ➤ It is the leading cause of disability in Americans under 45 years old
> ➤ About eight percent of low back pain becomes chronic
> ➤ Back pain is one of the leading causes of depression, divorce, drug addiction, and alcoholism
> ➤ Approximately 500,000 surgeries are performed yearly, yet only 20 percent are successful after a two-year period
> ➤ Over 100 billion dollars are spent yearly on the treatment of low back pain

The truly sad thing is that it doesn't have to be this way. People don't have to become so limited in their activities or debilitated by back pain. I can tell you that after treating literally thousands of people of all ages in my clinic over the last thirty-five years, fervently exploring all the leading-edge techniques (as well as employing those of my own discovery and invention), I have found nearly everyone – nearly *everyone* – can be helped to have a pain-free back without medication, and most often without surgery.

In fact, in my office today, eight out of ten new patients experience a significant improvement after their very first visit. What I've learned has literally transformed my practice and the lives of my patients, so trust that I know what I'm talking about.

Primary Focus

While some chiropractors expand their practices to include a range of ailments – from all kinds of structural issues to more holistic concerns such as wellness, weight loss, etc. – my concentration has always remained on the back. Why?

Back care is the singular area in which chiropractors can be the most effective and predictable out of all types of medical practitioners.

Very early in my career, I witnessed the importance of maintaining a healthy, strong, dependable back and recognized the particular capabilities of a chiropractor to accomplish just that. This is not to say that other practitioners cannot provide appropriate treatment for a person at other times - including even surgery in specific cases. Indeed, I will refer my own patients to other practitioners when I determine what they offer is better suited for a selected issue. That is why in this book, I will not limit the discussion only to what chiropractors can provide. I will address several other modalities of healing and what their practitioners bring, as well as the right circumstances or right timing to try them.

My intent is to educate readers to know:

- ➢ When to seek medical help for your back pain
- ➢ When it is best to see a chiropractor
- ➢ When it is time to try a different modality of treatment or perhaps leave one chiropractor and try another if you aren't seeing results
- ➢ When it is best to try physical therapy
- ➢ When you should consider surgery
- ➢ When *not* to head into surgery but try chiropractic and/or other non-invasive therapy at the same time
- ➢ When to consider epidurals along with your chiropractic/therapy care

This will be an easy-to-read book that offers a deeper understanding of when you should seek medical help for your condition, as well as prepare you to make the right decisions at a doctor's office, regardless of the type of practitioner you are seeing.

Remember: there is no better advocate for your well being than yourself! You simply need some "training." That is what this book will provide. In fact, you will find several images throughout these pages to better illustrate the concepts I am going to explain, as well as several integrated links to online videos that I've specifically created for this book. They demonstrate some of the techniques and treatments I describe, as well as simple exercises you can do to strengthen your back so you won't experience more back problems in the future. Please note that the videos are supplementary and not at all necessary to follow the information in this book; they are simply a visual for further clarification.

A Deeper Understanding To *Avoid* Back Issues

In addition to clearly explaining causes behind various types of back pain and the ways they may be treated, I will also illuminate many things you can immediately do for yourself to help *solve* and *avoid* back problems.

You will learn that the causes of back problems are most often not due to any deficiency in our inherent structure as humans, but due more to our actions – even common everyday activities that you might never have associated with back problems. One of the most notorious that we'll explore is the strain caused by *how* we sit. This has become more critical than ever as our culture has grown progressively more sedentary in our work, as well as our huge variety of entertainment that keeps us in front of computers or televisions for longer and longer periods. You'll see that today's causes of back pain can include other areas you might not have considered, such as the use of backpacks by students of all ages, to even the pandemic of texting that is causing its own set of spine-related issues.

More importantly than understanding the causes, you will discover how just by adjusting your daily activities *slightly*, you can make a *huge* difference in helping achieve a pain-free back. I've discovered these causes and modifications to activities after more than three decades of treating patients specifically for back pain.

My intention in writing this book is to bring hope, knowledge, and *results* to those of you who are dealing with back pain, regardless of its duration or severity. So please read on.

Regain your hope – and healthy back.

Chapter 2
Educated Patients

What You Don't Know *Can* Hurt You (Or At Least Won't Help)

A knowledgeable patient is essential when it comes to healing back pain - particularly low back pain. Why is this so critical? The reality is that 60 percent of all patients encountering back problems see their primary care physician for help. I'm not in any way disrespecting or belittling primary care physicians. They are extremely skilled and valuable in diagnosing and treating countless health issues. However, they do fall short with low back pain.

I work with numerous doctors, many of whom refer to me. Most of them readily acknowledge that they don't consider themselves experts in the treatment of low back pain. In truth, primary care physicians know little about how to *treat* back pain. The majority of patients are dismissed with having a muscle spasm and given an anti-inflammatory or a muscle relaxant. Treatment by medication alone often relieves or masks the symptoms of the problem rather than resolving the actual issue.

Equally unfortunate is that patients seldom question their medical doctor's appraisal. There's an assumption that doctors' orders are always correct. As a result, many patients with severe pain will get unnecessary surgery before they even try something like spinal decompression, chiropractic, physical therapy, or therapeutic exercises, all of which can resolve many types of back ailments. I've seen severe cases that looked like they needed surgery (even to me at first) that were healed with the proper decompression and treatment. However, most patients are never instructed to try it. Even worse, as indicated earlier, only 20 percent of spinal surgeries remain successful after the first two years; that means more surgery or more pain, or both. Also, many of the patients who would have improved prior to having surgery may not improve after surgery due to scar tissue, fusion, and other damage to the anatomy resulting from the surgery.

Regrettably, many primary care physicians once had less than optimal opinions regarding chiropractic and physical therapy. Fortunately, things have changed radically in the last ten years as more and more evidence points to chiropractic being the most successful mode of treatment for back pain. I now get referrals from many primary care physicians. Still, there are many physicians who completely bypass chiropractic and physical therapy. You should be aware of this bias so that you can explore other modes of treatment, even if your physician doesn't offer such a referral.

Please understand that I am not instructing you to avoid going to your primary care physician. I just want you to be fully informed of your options so you can determine the best course of action for *your* situation.

Different Types Of Treatment

It is also important for you as the patient to be aware of all the available treatment options, even when being treated by a chiropractor. In truth, there isn't any one standard of care when it comes to treating the back. This means that treatments can vary greatly from one chiropractic office to another. In fact, the approach that I've evolved over the years, which I will clarify later in this book, is an eclectic approach of many different modalities and professions.

Similarly, it is important to know when to switch from one approach or doctor to another if treatment isn't working. Patients are wonderfully loyal – some will stick with a doctor for years, even if their condition has yet to be resolved. Perhaps it is this tendency that has contributed to some people's belief that chiropractic didn't work for them, when changing to a chiropractor with a different approach could have done the trick.

An educated patient will be better able to judge the results they are (or are not) getting, as well as the treatment approach and recommendations coming their way.

Finding The Root Problem

When searching for the right practitioner, you must ask yourself: are they looking for and correcting the root cause of the problem? As said previously, physicians commonly prescribe medications to alleviate symptoms rather than dealing with the source of the problem. You may even encounter doctors who say that the majority of patients' problems are caused by emotional issues. They recommend stress reduction, meditation, and psychotherapy as a means to solve most back problems.

In reality, I'd agree that emotional stress can cause back problems (and probably believe that to a greater degree than most of my colleagues, orthopedists, and physical therapists). If you are experiencing fear, anger, or even grief, your muscles tend to contract in abnormal ways. If that continues long enough, these contractions can create uneven postures and cause misalignments in your back. Some doctors simply say to remove the sources of tension from your life, or give you medication to deal with your emotional stresses. With the back, even if the condition sourced from stress, if you have developed structural problems, you're going to have to deal with those as well. In fact, if it were true that one could resolve most back problems by simply dealing with emotional stress, I would have to consider myself a pretty good psychotherapist since eight out of ten of my patients improve significantly after their very first visit.

I would actually go further to also include environmental stresses as potential causes of misalignments. Exposure to harmful chemicals can overwhelm the nervous system, such that motor nerves imbalance muscles and create misalignments. These chemical exposures may come from pollution, products in our homes or in certain foods, as well as from alcohol or drugs (both recreational and prescription). Once these pollutants are recognized, you would be well advised to avoid further exposure while getting treatment to correct the back issues that have resulted. However, as is said in diagnostic classes, when you hear hoof beats, think of horses instead of zebras. Therefore, take the most likely cause before jumping to more remote conclusions.

Understanding The Cause

As stated in the prior chapter, back pain has sadly become an epidemic in our culture. Some attribute this significant increase as a reflection of our society growing older, with many baby boomers passing middle age. Yet, even this "logical" conclusion is over-simplified and even faulty. In fact, experiencing back pain is hardly confined to those growing older.

The truth is that back issues are occurring in younger and younger people. We are seeing increasing numbers of teenagers with back problems, and even children under ten showing symptoms of back-related issues.

Why is this happening?

While many of these issues (and their solutions) will be addressed in more detail in subsequent chapters, let me say now that much of this is happening because we are becoming a more sedentary culture. Across all age ranges, we are sitting more and exercising less. The amount of time we spend sitting in front of televisions, in front of computers at school, work, and home, and in the car as we commute longer distances in greater traffic is vastly increasing. *Sitting* is surprisingly one of the hardest positions on your back, particularly on your lumbar discs and sacroiliac joint. Sitting *improperly* magnifies the problem.

Children, in particular, are not exercising as often as even a few years ago when they would play ball after school, play tag, climb trees, or take part in other physical activities. Children are most often sitting in front of computers to the point where they literally have no physical activity at all. Even worse is that kids tend to wear heavy backpacks, especially for school as they carry numerous textbooks. This starts in elementary school and continues all the way through college. Young bodies are not built to carry such loads in this manner.

In a further development, there is now awareness of our culture's love of texting contributing to back issues for people of *all* ages. We, as humans, are designed to stand upright, but so many of us spend increasing amounts of time with our heads bent over a cellphone as we read and send text messages, causing physical stress and misalignment to our spine. When added up, many people could be spending hours every day in this unnatural position.

Yet another contributing factor to back problems is obesity, which is also reaching epidemic proportions, and at younger and younger ages. Carrying this extra weight adds physical stressors to our back.

Of course, there can be many other, often unexpected, causes behind back issues. For instance, pregnancy can cause back-related problems. Not only does pregnancy shift the gravity line in the low back area, causing more stress on the joints. It also prompts the body to release a hormone prior to birth to weaken the ligaments in the pelvis, particularly the sacroiliac joint, so that the pelvis can expand to facilitate birth. This is a key reason why many pregnant women will benefit from back treatment after giving birth.

All of this may be eye opening to you, as it has been to those of us in the healing profession. Unfortunately, I think we're going to continue seeing an increase in the number of low back (and even neck) problems due to many of these described behaviors and circumstances. But it doesn't have to be this way – and certainly doesn't have to be this way for you.

Do Not Give Up

A critical piece of advice I would give to patients is not to give up. All too often, people try some form of treatment for their back, find little improvement, and conclude that nothing can be done. They decide that they will just have to live with it, or that it's just part of growing older. However, just because a particular doctor or protocol failed doesn't mean you can't be helped. That would be like going to an Italian restaurant, not enjoying your meal and deciding you won't like other Italian restaurants. This particular restaurant just might not be the best one for you.

This is the importance of being an educated patient: to know there are other options.

With Knowledge, Hope Is Possible

To those of you who have tried a protocol with less than successful results (or haven't tried any), and have become resigned that you're simply going to have to live with back pain and all the limitations it places on your life – I am absolutely convinced that it doesn't have to be true. This is what motivated me to write this book. With over 30 years of experience, I've seen countless chronic conditions improve. In fact, no matter how bad your back is, recovery to some degree is possible – provided you get good, proper care.

Fortunately, that "good, proper care" has advanced considerably, even during my tenure of practice. There are many more options today than ever before, including from chiropractors like myself, that go far beyond simple manipulations and adjustments.

I think one reason some people are willing to live with their pain is that they believe the only choice they have is surgery. They might be frightened by the prospect, or have heard that it is often unsuccessful. Personally, I know that sometimes surgery *is* the only option for a patient, and when I recognize that, I refer them to surgeons I trust. But as I said earlier, the sad fact is that the majority of people getting back surgery today have never even tried treatments like spinal decompression. While spinal decompression has been around for some time, it too has advanced to a sophisticated degree as we have gained knowledge about how the body functions and heals.

Unfortunately, many *doctors* and patients are not educated on what's out there. While spinal decompression has become more common, the majority of chiropractic and physical therapy offices still do not employ it. As a result, spinal decompression is seldom suggested. Yet, it is a magnificent therapy – one where you'll typically know if it's helping within only a few treatments. I say this with confidence as we've been using spinal decompression in our office for 20 years.

My hope is that this book will not only inform patients about how to heal their own backs, but also encourage other chiropractors, physical therapists, and physicians to step out of their comfort zones and be open to expanding their protocols.

Chapter 3
Understanding Low Back Anatomy

The human body is astonishing. As a medical professional,
this is perhaps more apparent to me than most, as I
understand how its innumerable parts work together – and
heal together – given the right circumstances and support.

For the purpose of this chapter, I want readers to not only
comprehend low back anatomy, but also to really appreciate
it and take good care of it. The low back is comprised of the
pelvis, vertebrae, muscles, ligaments, tendons, nerves, and
discs. In addition, you should know that one of the primary
functions of the 24 vertebrae comprising the spinal column is
to house and protect the spinal cord, which extends down
from the brain. Through the vertical center of each vertebra
is an opening much like a doughnut. By stacking the 24
vertebrae on top of one another, these openings form a
tunnel – inside which is the spinal cord.

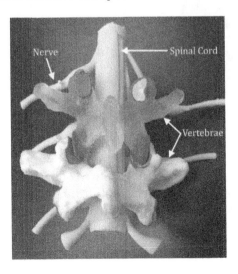

Being an extension of the brain, the spinal cord relays neurological impulses to all the different body areas (much like the electrical system in your home) via nerves. Located on both sides of each vertebra are additional small openings, which allow the nerves to exit the spinal cord. Between each vertebra is a sponge-like, jelly material called a disc, which acts as both a shock absorber *and* a fulcrum to allow each vertebra to move. These discs allow us to have mobility.

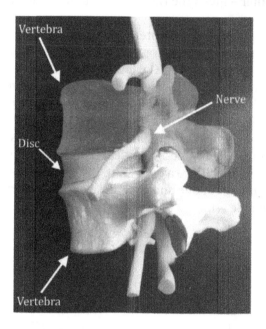

It is important to be aware of the positioning of the vertebrae in relation to these nerves, as back pain can be due to a misalignment of vertebrae such that they put *pressure* on these nerves. Another possible source of back pain is disc bulging or herniation, which result from the jelly causing the back portion of the disc to balloon outward, therefore placing abnormal pressure on the spinal cord and/or spinal nerves.

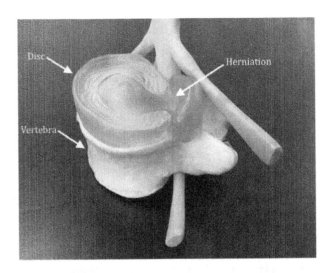

The entire spine sits on top of the pelvis, which is formed by the sacrum and the right and left ilia. Where the sacrum and the ilium meet is called the sacroiliac joint.

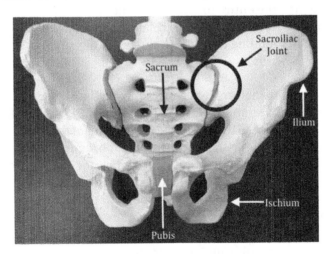

The sacroiliac is a very tight, weight-bearing joint with little flexibility or pliability. It allows us to stand for extended periods of time without fatigue or pain, provided the sacroiliac joint is intact. As we'll learn, we can experience pain when the sacroiliac joint is out of alignment. Medical studies have shown that of the three positions – standing, lying, and sitting – sitting by far causes the greatest pressure and stress on the lumbar discs and sacroiliac joints. In fact, in developing nations where sitting is not as prevalent as it is in the United States, the amount of back problems is substantially reduced. I will address sitting and its effects on back pain in more detail in chapter 11.

Interestingly, between discs and sacroiliac joints, discs are the most agreed upon cause for back pain. The sacroiliac joint, on the other hand, is a much more controversial area. Some professionals state that it seldom relates to back pain, while others claim it is the ultimate cause of most back pain. After treating back pain for 30 years, my opinion is that sacroiliac disorders are a formidable equal to lumbar discs in terms of being a source of pain. Once subluxated – or out of alignment – the entire foundation of the spine becomes compromised, producing abnormal pressure on the soft tissues surrounding the vertebrae, such as ligaments, tendons, and discs.

To complicate matters further, stabilizing the SI (sacroiliac) joint can be as simple as it is difficult, to nearly impossible at times. Fortunately, thanks to the integration of different professions along with the advancement of support and new technologies in chiropractic, the prognosis for stabilization is much better. Additionally, in most cases, the SI and a disc bulge or herniation frequently respond to the same form of therapy, as we will later describe in more detail. So even with some "controversy" about which is the cause, both can sometimes benefit from the same treatment.

Now, let's dive deeper so we understand the reasons behind the high frequency of low back pain.

Chapter 4

Understanding The Causes
Of Low Back Pain

As I've pointed out, back pain is one of the most prevalent medical problems facing America today, and it's only increasing. One out of every three people will seek professional help at one point in their lives to deal with back pain. Try to think of another medical condition that encompasses so many people (aside from, perhaps, dental cavities).

The specific cause of back pain will vary from patient to patient, and finding the true cause is essential to proper treatment. Unfortunately, while this would appear to be obvious, the type of treatment that patients receive will too often be a function of what is favored by the particular professional they visit, which may or may not be the most suitable for their condition. In fact, the most consistently used forms of treatment come from the primary care physician (mainly medication), and their typical goal is to relieve the patient of pain. That is not a bad goal to have, but it doesn't solve the problem or prevent the present condition from reoccurring or worsening. That is one reason why typical back conditions – widespread as they may be – are still often a mystery to those experiencing them. So let me pose a question here that I am sometimes asked, which will launch us into understanding back conditions:

Is a pain-free back necessarily a healthy back?

A genuinely healthy back is one where the vertebrae, discs, hips, muscles, and other supportive tissues all function in their proper synergistic relationship with each other. That's why the simple absence of pain is absolutely *not* true criteria for a healthy back.

This is the unfortunate flaw in the preferred treatment consisting of anti-inflammatories, muscle relaxants, and painkillers. Eighty percent of these patients will feel better in one week, only to falsely assume that they are back to normal. The imbalance that produced the pain and brought them to the doctor in the first place still exists. That's why a high percentage of these patients will experience a reoccurrence of their problem, usually with an increased severity.

True Back Conditions

To educate and take away the mystery behind back pain, I want to build upon the last chapter and further describe the specific medical conditions causing low back pain, as well as put them in the order of which occurs most commonly in people.

To start off, I can tell you right away from having worked with thousands of patients' backs over the years that the top two leading causes of low back problems are disc herniations and sacroiliac joint issues.

Herniated Discs

Our vertebrae each have a sponge-like cushion called a disc that separates one bone from another. Inside each disc is a small jelly center. Disc herniation is when this jelly breaks through the outer layer of the disc, or annulus, and into the space where it puts pressure on the nerve tissue.

Because people sit often, which causes pressure on the disc to increase in general, that jelly can begin to break down the disc, typically from the inside out. The disc wall then starts to balloon, which is a bulging disc. Eventually, the jelly can actually begin to bleed out, and that's when you start to get a herniated disc.

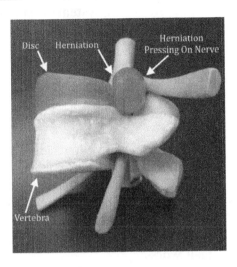

Sensations from a disc herniation can vary. Some people feel numbness and others feel tingling. Some may feel burning, while others feel pain. Regardless of the symptoms you may experience, this condition is one of the most common causes of back problems – and many people have it without realizing it.

How is that possible? If you put pressure on a nerve, it can cause pain. If the disc bulges but doesn't place pressure on the nerve, it may create some instability in the back but may not create any pain whatsoever. In fact, if you were to take MRIs of the population that is not experiencing back pain at all, 30 percent would still have herniated discs. Many people simply don't know it because the herniation is not putting any pressure on the nerve. This is another reason why lack of pain doesn't necessarily mean a healthy back.

What about those who *do* notice something? One of the common symptoms of a herniation is pain radiating down one side – it can travel into the buttocks and into the leg. The pain can also travel down the back, side, or front of the leg. Each nerve has a different wiring system extending to different parts of the leg, so depending on the location of the herniation, it will impact different aspects of a nerve and affect different parts of the leg. It is very unusual for a herniation to be on both sides, though it can be.

Some common signals indicating a disc herniation:

- The body is slightly tilted sideways
- Symptoms are typically worse in the morning and alleviate as the day goes on
- Getting out of bed and putting on shoes in the morning are difficult
- Walking usually feels better, and sitting often feels worse
- It is painful to sit

An MRI will confirm if there is a disc herniation, as well as show if the disc is putting pressure on the nerve. The chiropractor can then determine if the symptoms are related to that nerve pressure.

https://youtu.be/unMRbUrzEpQ

Sacroiliac Joint Dysfunction – More Common Than Realized

As previously described, the sacroiliac joints are the two joints in the low back at the base of the spine that attach the ilia (that support the hipbones) to the sacrum. The sacrum is the platform on which the spinal column sits. It's a strong joint that should be held together very tightly, but if misaligned or strained, it will cause pain in the low back. Pain can radiate into the groin, thigh, buttocks area, hip area, and/or down the front of the leg above the knee. Once the sacroiliac joint actually separates, it can be difficult to get it back into place again. It is possible, but can be difficult.

https://youtu.be/FyhSGNCUq8s

Because this joint dysfunction can mimic a disc problem and causes radiating pain into the legs, most doctors assume it's a type of nerve impingement from a disc. So, for many people, the sacroiliac joint may be the most perplexing joint in the body when it comes to back pain. Even in professions dealing with back problems, there is great variation on how much emphasis is put on this area. I would say that chiropractors pay more attention than most, and it's certainly my own experience that the SI (sacroiliac) joint is a major player when it comes to low back problems. I've seen it proven clinically in my practice over and over again. Though frequently overlooked, the SI joint dysfunction is actually far more common than most doctors realize.

Unfortunately, diagnostic tests generally do not detect it. Neither X-rays nor MRIs will show it, but it can produce severe levels of low back pain. However, with the patient lying on their back, this condition appears to produce a leg that is functionally longer on the side with pain 80 percent of the time.

Here are a few other symptoms that indicate that you may have a sacroiliac dysfunction:

- The pain itself can feel like a throbbing toothache-like sensation
- Walking up or down stairs seems to increase the pain
- Generally, your back pain seems to be localized to one side, and the pain can radiate into the groin
- Transitioning from a seated position to a standing position can be very painful
- Once seated, you tend to prefer putting more weight on one side of your buttocks than the other
- Placing more weight on one leg while standing seems to help
- When looking in the mirror, one hip bone seems higher than the other

So, how does one end up with SI joint dysfunction? It can be a result of traumas, ranging from the subtle strain from stepping off a curb or step unexpectedly to a whiplash-type injury. It can also slowly evolve from poor posture and/or poor ergonomics, especially while sitting. Regardless of how your back pain started, applying the protocols that help with SI dysfunction, including home exercises that I detail later in this book, will help you move in a direction of increased abilities and decreased discomfort.

Spinal Stenosis

Spinal stenosis is a narrowing of the spinal canal. This can result from a congenitally (something you're born with) narrow spinal canal, and/or can be caused by bone spurs (a form of spinal arthritis) that begin to lip into the spinal canal space. Spinal stenosis is more common in the elderly, though it is not a natural part of aging.

To better understand this condition, imagine you're going into New York City from New Jersey through the Lincoln Tunnel. It is one to two miles long and only two lanes.

Imagine there is nobody else in the tunnel and you have to drive your car sixty miles an hour from one end to the other. Could you do it without hitting the sides of the tunnel? Inevitably everyone says absolutely. No problem.

Now imagine the tunnel much narrower – its sides are only six to eight inches away from your car on either side, and now you have to drive sixty miles an hour without touching the sides of the walls. That's spinal stenosis. There is definitely room for the spinal cord, but there is not much forgiveness.

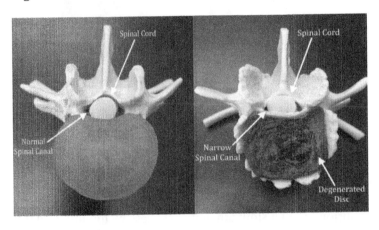

In the body – getting in any "wrong" position or even standing upright can actually cause the canal to put pressure on the nerves. What "opens up" the canal and increases the interior dimension is sitting. That's why sitting is more comfortable for people with this condition.

Aside from spinal stenosis, you can also have *foraminal stenosis*. This is when there is a narrowing of the small openings, or vertebral foramen, where the nerves come out of the vertebra on each side of the spine. How does this happen? Sometimes people have genetically smaller openings, but in other cases, as the discs begin to wear away and lose some vertical height, the openings close.

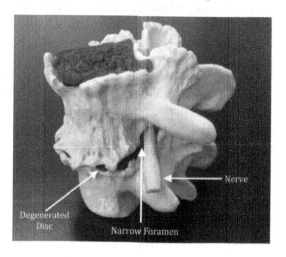

Typically, these stenotic conditions are seen in patients as they get older, usually 60 years of age and older. As they are progressive conditions, they usually result from years of inactivity. The more active people are, the higher the probability that they will not have the full effects of spinal stenosis. While that's not an absolute, you can help the condition or even slow down its progress by maintaining a certain level of exercise.

It's important to understand that the more you stretch and have motion in a body area, the more likely that that area will not become arthritic, or at least not become abnormally arthritic. In fact, studies have been performed on animals where a completely healthy joint was immobilized. After six months of immobility, the beginning stages of arthritis had already begun. So my advice to you – move!

What are the noticeable symptoms of spinal stenosis?

- Usually discomfort, numbness, or tingling in both legs
- Sitting provides relief, as do bent legs
- Walking becomes tiring very quickly
- Lying in bed feels best
- Symptoms are best in the mornings and progressively worsen as the day goes on

Therefore, an older person with tingling, numbness, or pain in both legs who prefers sitting, who will tire if they walk for more than five minutes, and has to sit to give themselves relief, likely has some form of stenosis. This diagnosis can be confirmed with an MRI, which can also help determine the type of stenosis.

Degenerative Disc Disease

It is important to realize that this is not an actual disease. It is more of a condition when the discs – the small cushions between vertebrae made up of mostly fluid – begin to deteriorate.

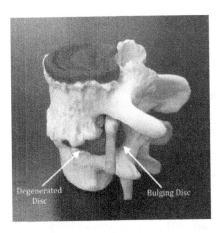

The discs of a young person are at the height of the amount of fluid, making for very spongy and flexible tissue. With age, trauma, and inactivity, the discs begin to lose fluid and start to dry out. A healthy disc is like a plum – as it begins to degenerate, it turns into a raisin.

One of the effects of degenerative disc disease is that it can lead to foraminal spinal stenosis; the compressed channels narrow the small openings where the nerves come out from the vertebrae on each side of the spine. With degenerative disc disease, you also get an arthritic condition of the joint. This happens when the joint becomes unstable and the body tries to fuse the joints together, a mechanism in the body to try to protect and stabilize itself.

Pinched Nerves

You will frequently hear patients state that they think they have a pinched nerve. In reality, a pinched nerve is not a condition, but rather a result of abnormal pressure on one of the spinal nerves, which results in pain. The most common causes are:

- Misaligned vertebra
- Disc herniation
- Spinal stenosis
- Foraminal stenosis
- Disc degeneration

Sciatica

While this is a word many people have heard, it also isn't a "condition" so much as an effect. Sciatica is essentially another name for a pinched nerve. The difference is that sciatica is an impingement of the sciatic nerve – the last nerve coming out of the last segment of the spine – which travels through the pelvis and down the back of your leg to the foot. It is actually the largest nerve in your body.

The most common causes of sciatica are the same as those found with other pinched nerves. Although the majority of sciatica is caused by disc herniation, it can also be due to foraminal spinal stenosis, misalignment, or simply the joint hitting the nerve.

Regardless of the cause, sciatica creates an inflammation of this last nerve, which can cause pain in your low back and down your leg.

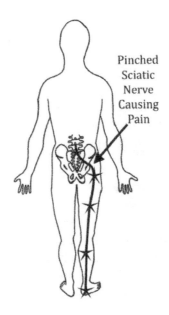

Pinched
Sciatic
Nerve
Causing
Pain

Spondylolisthesis

Spondylolisthesis can be caused by a birth defect in which part of the vertebra doesn't fuse together, and so the front and back portions of the vertebra begin to separate. It affects about three to five percent of the population and the majority of cases occur in the very last vertebra – identified as L-5 (lumbar 5). It is divided into four categories of severity:

grades one through four, and fortunately, the majority of cases are at a grade one, which has no effect on the body and causes no pain whatsoever, provided the condition is stable.

The key factor in whether the condition is a problem is if the spondylolisthesis is stable or unstable. What you want is to have your doctor order a flexion/extension X-ray. That means an X-ray is taken while you bend backward at your low back (extension) and again as you bend forward (flexion).

Taking pictures in this manner will help show if the spondylolisthesis is unstable – that is, if the vertebra starts to shift position (normally, it should not) from movement. If it is unstable, that could be a cause of back pain. A series of very specific exercises would then be prescribed for the patient to assist with their condition. Severe instability of the L-5 vertebra as a result of the spondylolisthesis may require surgical intervention to stabilize.

Scoliosis

Another commonly described condition is scoliosis, which is abnormal "side bending" of the spine. It is mostly seen in children – especially girls – usually at the beginning of puberty and coming to its maximum distortion as one approaches adulthood. This is normally checked in school, but can be overlooked.

It is best discovered early. We had one case with a woman from Allendale Township that was overlooked by the school system and her parents. By the time she came to us, she was about 30 years old with a curvature of 54 degrees. Unfortunately, once the curvature gets to this level, surgery is needed to put a rod into the body from one vertebra to another; otherwise the spine can literally collapse on itself.

Parents should be aware to keep an eye on the spine as their children grow. You do this simply by standing behind the child and having them bend forward to touch their toes while you look to see if one side mounds more than the other.

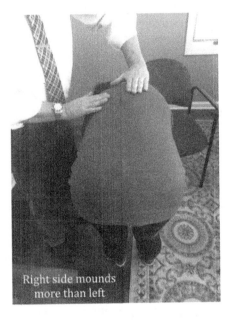

Right side mounds more than left

If they do have an abnormal curvature, then take the child to someone who specializes in scoliosis to X-ray the area and measure the degree of side curvature. Provided the curvature is relatively small, the key is to determine if it's progressive. One could have a curvature of fourteen degrees and live a healthy life. But if the curvature is growing at a significant rate at such a young age, like one degree each month, then it is advisable to find an orthopedist who specializes in scoliosis in order to brace it – that is, have the patient wear an external brace. It would be worn during their growth phase and at some point would no longer be needed. While the child will likely not be thrilled about this, the biggest problem with scoliosis is once it becomes severe and structurally unsound. As the scoliosis progresses, the ribs attached to the vertebra can put pressure on the lungs and heart, which becomes the greatest danger.

Provided you catch and brace it in time, serious problems can be prevented in most cases of scoliosis. Fortunately, most incidences aren't so severe and simply need to be observed and supported with a home exercise program specifically for scoliosis.

Idiopathic Back Pain

Idiopathic back pain is just another name for back pain with an unknown cause. Although this is not that common (at least, not in our office), it is a condition that shows up every so often. In such cases, the cause of the back problem may indeed be emotional. Now, this is not to say that this patient is a malingerer or a faker at all. The fact that the pain is caused by an emotional issue does not mean the patient is not feeling pain. The solution can be as simple as the patient getting something off their chest, or getting some professional help. It's been recognized that holding in intense emotions without expressing them can negatively affect your health in many ways. As Woody Allen once said, "I don't get angry, I grow a tumor instead."

Interestingly, idiopathic back pain doesn't seem to follow any particular pattern like a patient with a disc herniation or stenosis. When asked if the pain gets worse with walking or sitting too long, the patient with spinal stenosis will say it hurts to walk and it feels good to sit, while the patient with the disc herniation will say just the opposite. But the patient with idiopathic back pain doesn't seem to be able to identify any particular pattern. Again, that doesn't mean it is not real.

Chapter 5

Flexion vs. Extension: Which Type Of Patient Are You?

Regardless of whether you have spinal stenosis, disc degeneration, or sacroiliac dysfunction, you basically fall into one of two categories in terms of therapeutic approaches and exercises that will best serve your recovery and strengthening: flexion or extension.

Yet, many doctors and even chiropractors won't discuss this with you! Fortunately, YOU can determine if you're a flexion or extension type patient. Although there are many types of back diagnoses, the key to getting better is determining whether to incorporate flexion (forward bending) types of exercises or extension (backward bending) types of exercises.

Of the two types, extension is more ideal. A young spine is a spine that can extend backward and it is preferable to have this ability. People who have lost this ability are further from having a healthy back than someone who can extend their back. Regardless of your age, the inability to extend is a sign of an older back. Do know that there are many young people for whom bending backward during the initial phases of treatment will cause irritation. This in no way indicates an "old back." It is simply that the inflammation in the disc area may initially be too great to bend backward.

A patient profile should include determining in which of the two categories you belong. Below are some simple criteria for each:

Flexion Type Patient

- Typically 60 years and older
- Usually exhibits poor posture
- In general, bending backward is difficult and somewhat uncomfortable
- MRI shows stenosis or some type of disc and/or joint degeneration
- Can experience paresthesia (abnormal tingling or pain in lower extremities) in one or both legs
- Pain or discomfort is usually chronic and has been getting progressively worse
- Back pain lessens while sitting
- Walking worsens back pain, requiring frequent rests due to discomfort
- Walking longer distances becomes more difficult, progressively getting worse over time
- Lying on the back with legs bent with a pillow under the knees feels best
- Mornings are usually better, discomfort worsens throughout day
- Progress is usually very slow and seldom is there dramatic improvement

Extension Type Patient

- Typically are teens to 59 years of age
- MRI shows some type of disc bulge or herniation
- X-rays may be negative (meaning no problem is found)
- The upper body posture can be tilting to one side
- Can experience pain down the leg – usually the back of the leg and almost always only one leg
- Back pain feels worse while sitting
- Standing and walking are more comfortable

- Transitional movements such as going from sitting to standing produces discomfort or pain
- Mornings are usually worse; once up you are somewhat better
- Coughing and/or sneezing usually irritates the low back area
- In the acute phase, bending backward may cause sudden sharp pain
- Improvement can be dramatic, where patients could feel 100 percent better by the end of the day, only to regress back to zero the next morning

When looking at the above two categories, keep in mind that not all of the indications must apply to you. Yet, you should be able to sense with a good level of certainty that you fit into one of the categories.

Let me assist further by offering different scenarios for these two categories that put many of these symptoms together. Read the following two descriptions and ask yourself which scenario matches you more closely. Most cases never accurately reflect any individual 100 percent, but what you are experiencing will show a good number of similarities to one of these examples.

You also need to ask yourself to what *degree* of severity you fit into the scenarios described below. The degree of severity will determine *the gradient* – that is, how quickly and aggressively at which we would approach a back exercise program that is appropriate for your condition.

Flexion Scenario

You are a 65 years or older male or female who is not overly active. You spend a good amount of time sitting: either reading, watching TV, or at the computer. In fact, sitting is generally the most comfortable position for you. Overall, your back problem came on slowly and subtly and has gradually worsened. Your pain feels better in the morning and seems to progressively worsen during the day, sometimes leading to the need to lie down, or at least sit, to get some relief. Doing extended shopping or walking has become more challenging, and sitting periodically while shopping or just being out is helpful in relieving your back problem. You feel the pain across the low back and it sometimes travels into the lower extremities – one leg, or even both. The feeling you experience in the lower legs can be tingling, burning, or crawling and does not always have to be painful. You have noticed that the amount of time you are able to stand and/or walk between rest periods is slowly but progressively getting shorter. If you're a golfer, it is getting more and more difficult to walk the entire 18 holes, or you have no choice but to use a golf cart.

Of everything just mentioned, the *key* indicators for being a flexion patient are:

- The older you are, the higher probability that you fall into the flexion program
- The more inactive you are, the greater probability for being a flexion patient
- The frequency of having to sit after walking or standing is also a strong indication of falling into the flexion scenario

The more you agree with the three areas just mentioned, the greater probability that you have a flexion scenario, and the more you will need to start exercises off at a slower pace or gradient.

Extension Scenario

You are younger than 60 years old and have developed a back problem usually after a certain activity. The onset could have resulted from simply bending over, lifting a newspaper, brushing your teeth, or sneezing, or a day or two after lifting a relatively heavy object. You are a relatively active person and this condition has interfered or become a nuisance with doing activities that you like. As the day goes on, it seems to get better. Yet, come morning, it seems like you've lost whatever ground you gained from the previous day. In fact, getting out of bed is difficult and putting on your shoes is just as challenging. Once you are on your feet and walking, the pain seems to diminish. The pain is in the low back, sometimes on one side, and can radiate into the buttocks and leg area, typically on one side of the body. Driving the car is a painful experience, as is getting through your workday if you do a lot of sitting. Coughing and sneezing increase the pain, as can having a bowel movement. You feel best lying on your side, and in most cases, with the painful side up. Pain can be local to the low back area, or can travel all the way to the foot, usually on one side only.

If after reading this scenario, you agree that this fits your profile more than the flexion program, you would proceed with the extension program. I include safe and effective exercise protocols in a later chapter for both flexion and extension conditions.

Professional Help

Let me reinforce that what I've presented in terms of classifying yourself is in no way a replacement for sound professional exams and testing. There is no substitute for getting expert help when it comes to back pain, regardless if you have a flexion or an extension problem. However, better understanding of your back pain and the different treatments available will make you an educated patient. That is doubly important, because regardless of all the technology that a professional uses to help diagnose the cause of back pain, *what the patient tells the doctor may still be the most important part of the evaluation.* Therefore, the categorizations given here should not only help guide you as a patient trying to determine which exercise protocol may help, but also give you an idea of what is important to tell your healthcare professional. And here is something very important to know, especially if you've been trying unsuccessfully to improve your back for some time:

Finding the proper program and therapy is exceedingly effective as a rule.

With over 35 years of experience, I can say with complete certainty that if you were to take 1000 patients who were recommended surgery after trying therapy and were to actually find their true diagnosis (and apply the proper treatment for that diagnosis), *at least* 80 percent of those patients would see a significant improvement.

I really want to emphasize this again: as complicated as back problems can be, at least 80 to 90 percent of the population of back sufferers will show a considerable degree of progress by first determining the right category they fall into, and then approaching that category's treatment and particular exercises *with the correct gradient.* By that I mean a patient at 85 years of age, for example, needs to start off at a significantly slower pace than a 70-year-old patient when doing a flexion program.

I will also point out that regardless of whether you are in a flexion program or an extension program, small intervals of exercises, somewhere between five and ten minutes done two to three times a day, will provide better results than doing one 45 minute program once a day. That idea sometimes goes against the general mindset in this country of "more, more, more" – that if a little is good, a lot is even better. It is simply not true with healing backs. It also makes *doing* the exercises more manageable and more likely to take place, as there's no large single block of time required. Additionally, since I am not there to guide you, I want you to err on the side of caution; this will better help you make solid, *lasting* progress with back care.

I'm taking the time to clearly define these flexion and extension categories, as they are so important to your healing that I refer to these two groupings in various chapters throughout the book, particularly in chapter 17, which focuses on the *proper* illustrated exercises to help both categories of people improve their backs.

Chapter 6
Not All Chiropractors
Are The Same

Chiropractic has evolved throughout the years, and the adjustments used to realign vertebrae have become gentler and more specific in most offices. Chiropractors require a pre-medical degree and an additional four years of schooling quite similar to medical doctors, but with more emphasis placed on spinal mobilization and less on the study of pharmacology. Even though all are highly trained, not all chiropractors are the same, and chiropractic approaches and techniques can vary from office to office.

There are different types of philosophies regarding how to practice. Some chiropractors believe that their main priority is to find subluxations (vertebrae that are misaligned) and realign them. This is what is called a subluxation-based practice. Many chiropractors will follow this model of practice; the basic belief being that the body does not need further medications or surgeries provided it is free of nerve interference caused by misaligned vertebrae. The body knows how to heal itself when there is no such nerve impingement.

The subluxation-based practice is one where the Doctor of Chiropractic will educate you regarding subluxations and will recommend a series of adjustments to correct any subluxations. Once these subluxations have been corrected, patients are recommended to go on a support or maintenance program to maintain the state of being subluxation free. Millions of patients see these chiropractors and are additionally on what many chiropractors call "a wellness program."

Focus On The Low Back

In every field, there are practitioners who decide to dedicate themselves to particular types of problems. While chiropractic in general offers very effective remedies to a wide range of physical ailments, I decided twenty years ago to move away from the subluxation-based practice and into a condition-based practice. I decided to dedicate my chiropractic ability toward specializing in the treatment of low back pain and low back-related leg pain. I am not alone in this approach, but will admit that you will have to look a little harder to find someone who specializes in this manner.

In my case, I eventually developed the ability to get eight out of ten back patients significantly better after their first visit – whether it was by realigning misaligned vertebrae, getting a disc that was bulging against a nerve back into place, or by using decompression to hydrate a disc and reduce pressure on a nerve. I am in no way implying that how I practice is unilaterally better than a chiropractor with a subluxation-based practice. The big difference is that in my practice, getting low back symptoms better is the priority, whereas the priority of a subluxation-based practice is removing subluxations and maintaining wellness.

I cite this so that you know my point of view behind what I'm conveying in this book. It may already be obvious to you since my emphasis throughout is strongly on the lower back, which is where most back problems are or originate.

Ask your chiropractor about his or her practice philosophy. If it is a subluxation-based practice and the doctor informs you that their job is not dealing with symptoms, but to free the body of subluxation – that's fine. But if your symptoms do not improve in a relatively short time, you may want to try another chiropractic office. The truth is that the body's ability to heal and respond to care when a pinched nerve (due to a disc herniation or a misaligned joint or vertebrae) becomes freed is remarkable. Although the chiropractor may be adjusting you, he may be missing where the true interference is – and that's where your symptoms provide valuable feedback.

In my office, if I am on adjustment three or four and the patient still hasn't felt any improvement, I am certainly going to reevaluate and change my approach because the body really does respond that fast, and I am obviously not getting to the core of the problem. You shouldn't need a year of care to clear your problem – the body is more extraordinary than that. My belief is that if you're treated by a chiropractor or PT and a couple of weeks go by with no improvement, and they don't make the effort to change his or her formula and approach, that's an indication that something is missing and it might be time to look for new help.

My Path To Treating Low Backs

As I said, over twenty years ago I had a subluxation-based office. I educated patients on the principles of chiropractic and maintained a very large, strong practice. I wasn't focused specifically on symptoms, but really on freeing subluxations. But that began shifting as I started to learn that there are *many* techniques that can help open a pinched nerve if you find out exactly how it is being pinched. I came to realize that in low back cases – provided you *truly* get to the cause of the problem and apply the correct technique to undo the nerve impingement – most people get better, and in most cases, very quickly.

This experience is what prompted me to change from subluxation-based to what I call a more condition-based practice. I began the shift by placing more responsibility on the symptoms and whether or not somebody was getting better. Since I became a symptom-oriented doctor, the results have been extraordinary and my practice has actually prospered far beyond how it had previously. Again, this may be something you wish to question a prospective chiropractor about as you consider being treated.

Another question you might ask could be in regards to the "technology" they use in their office. Most people think of chiropractors doing all their work with just their hands. That can be true for many, and it has delivered proven results over many years. However, some chiropractors do employ certain technologies that were developed to yield truly phenomenal results and provide truly leading-edge treatments specifically for low back pain sufferers.

In the next four chapters, we will look at some of those technological breakthroughs, specifically relating to low backs. These technologies can be incredibly valuable in healing low backs, and at a much faster pace when utilized by a skilled chiropractor. Even with all the innovations I have seen in recent times, there is still nothing as important to helping a patient get better as the chiropractor's experience and knowledge of how and when to incorporate these new technologies.

Chapter 7
Spinal Decompression

I can absolutely say the technological advances that have occurred over the last 15 years have truly been a Godsend for many back pain sufferers. This chapter covers one of the most effective technologies for treating backs to which I unhesitatingly give five stars. In all my years of practice, no equipment has gone so far beyond my expectations as the spinal decompression system.

Spinal decompression is essentially a form of computerized traction specifically designed to treat disc herniations. In the body, each vertebra is separated by a disc, which has a jelly center. Factors such as trauma, excessive or improper lifting, or extended periods of sitting can cause the jelly center to break through the surrounding wall in which it is encapsulated and bulge out, putting abnormal pressure onto the spinal cord or the nerve roots as they leave the spine.

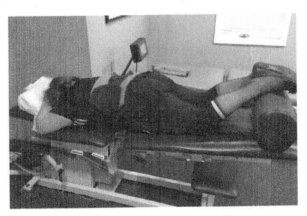

Spinal decompression produces a "negative gravity" at the disc level. A negative gravity creates a suction or vacuum on the disc material, causing the jelly that is protruding outward to be naturally pulled or sucked back inward and away from the nerve.

Interestingly, many years ago, patients with severe episodes of acute back pain were put in hospitals and harnessed in steady traction for six to eight hours a day for up to ten days with a heavy heated grain sack placed on their back. As you might imagine, even though it often achieved results, this traction fell out of favor and is still considered by some as a questionable treatment for back problems.

Yet today, almost every one of the more advanced back centers will have spinal decompression – which is essentially a highly sophisticated and evolved form of traction. It doesn't hold a continuous traction as was done long ago. Instead, it incorporates computerization to create intermittent traction lasting just 10 to 30 seconds at a time for a certain amount of cycles, depending on what the practitioner wants. An entire treatment can vary anywhere from eight to twenty minutes. We have clearly come a long way from the eight-hour static traction protocols.

I have had the privilege of working with computerized spinal decompression therapy now for more than 15 years, and I can say without any reservations that spinal decompression is the gold standard for treating back problems associated with disc disorders.

As a result, today if you are at a pain point where you need help, hospital care may not be the best choice, other than getting some medication to help relieve pain, reduce inflammation, or decrease muscle spasms. Back centers specializing in and equipped to deal with low back disc disorders, stenosis, and sciatica will, in most cases, be a significantly better choice. We have had many cases that even I initially thought would need surgery that were turned around by spinal decompression.

I don't often have the good fortune of ordering a second MRI for a patient after treatment is complete (as most times insurance won't cover another if it is not directly tied to surgery), but I have had patients whose second MRI confirms that the disc has been completely restored back to normal after having spinal decompression.

Who Would Benefit From Spinal Decompression?

Spinal decompression therapy is designed for rehabilitation of the spinal disc. Good candidates are patients with the following conditions: herniated discs, degenerative disc disease, spinal stenosis, sciatica, tingling and numbness in the arms and legs, or degenerative joint disease.

Are There Contraindications Or Side Effects?

Patients with fused low backs or who have metal screws or plates in their spines should not have spinal decompression therapy. Also, patients with severe degrees of osteoporosis are best served to stay away from this modality.

Even though these are the only contraindications, patients receiving spinal decompression therapy may experience some spinal discomfort following the therapy. This is normal and not severe, though may last up to 24 hours.

However, an important note to patients – and doctors: a side reaction sometimes occurs to those receiving spinal decompression for the first time that's nicknamed the *traction reaction*. This can be a severe spasm at the end of the session, which can be quite alarming to the patient.

Fortunately this reaction is usually over in 15 to 30 minutes, though in very rare cases can last through the next day. If it does occur, it almost always will happen only in the first session. No lasting harm is done, though the spasm can be quite intense. The saddest thing is that no matter how much the patient may need the decompression therapy, convincing them to continue treatment after this is often nearly impossible.

Fortunately, over the years of practice, my office has completely eliminated this severe reaction. However, it can happen with many doctors, especially newer chiropractors who tend to think that if a little pull is good, more pull is better. Doctors need to be aware that patients with disc disorders who also have an SI component are more likely to have a traction reaction. Doctors have to be very slow with applying pressure to the patient, and slow when removing the belts from around the patient.

Spinal decompression is such a valuable treatment that you don't want the patient to give up the opportunity to continue with it. That's why a doctor should err on the side of being very light – especially on the first visit. Once you get past the first visit, the patient should be fine and there shouldn't be any reaction, which is why we're especially cautious in our office with the first appointment.

The main point of telling you this is that as a patient, you should be proactive in your treatment – by insisting to the doctor that you want your first visit to be very gentle.

It should be recognized that at the conclusion of any spinal decompression session, there is some instability in the area. This makes sense, as you've just spent time pulling on the area to expand the vertebrae apart. That instability is why you want to do some walking after decompression to help stabilize it again. In our office, we have patients walk on a treadmill for ten minutes with good posture – breast bone high – with the addition of ice on their back. What's *not* a good idea is to just get in your car and go home at the conclusion of decompression. You should at least walk briefly on a treadmill or, if there is no treadmill, walk around the block and come back into the office so they can double check that all is well before you leave (an example is examining to ensure your leg lengths are extending equally).

How Many Sessions Are Needed And Are They Covered By Insurance?

The recommended program for disc rehabilitation can vary from patient to patient, depending on the severity of the disc disorder. Most patients will experience relief within the first five sessions. After the fifth decompression session, patient treatment is reevaluated to determine how many, if any, additional decompressions are necessary. It is often recommended that patients with degenerative conditions such as degenerative joint disease, degenerative disc disease, or spinal stenosis, but who have done well with spinal decompression, should stay on a maintenance program of once a week to once a month, depending on the severity of their condition. Again, each circumstance is different.

There are some centers that follow a generic approach with decompression, which is to offer a set number of visits for a set dollar amount, independent of your particular condition and situation. I would recommend a patient confronted with this situation to consider a different office, where a set "per visit fee" is charged instead, depending on your insurance. Decompression has a billable insurance code and is, in fact, covered.

For those patients who do not have insurance, I would recommend they consider prepaying at most five to ten visits at a time, and after each interval, evaluate how they are doing. I've had cases I thought would respond well to decompression, only to decide after five sessions that we should go in a different direction. In reality, patients in our office are told to expect some symptomatic improvement in three to five visits, but if we do not see progress at the end of five visits, the patient will be reevaluated to determine a change in the course of action.

Is Spinal Decompression The Only Care Needed?

As I previously mentioned, spinal decompression rehabilitates the disc itself, which produces fast, effective results for back and leg pain sufferers. However, in my opinion, pre- and post-therapy such as stretching, muscle energy technique, and exercises to strengthen your core (abdominal muscles) are necessary in order to obtain maximum results (which may not be standard in all offices).

Are There Different Types Of Spinal Decompression Systems?

There are actually many different types of spinal decompression systems, all claiming to have an advantage over their competitors. In fact, many patients have come to my office asking if I was aware of the DRX 9000 and if I had that equipment. The DRX 9000 is by far the most advertised decompression program and will do what it is advertised to do, which is to decompress the disc tissue. However, there are newer and more advanced table systems, on which patients can be decompressed not only on the back (called supine), but also facing down (prone) and on their sides. In fact, the more sophisticated decompression tables allow the chiropractor to apply any of 54 different table positions that will maximize the chances for the disc material to return to its normal position.

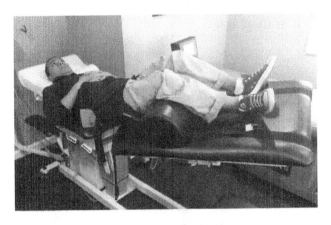

The VPADD

One system we particularly like is called the VPADD, which is an acronym for Vertical Pneumatic Axial Disc Decompression. The name and protocol were actually developed by me about 15 years ago. The VPADD is a better choice for patients who we believe are in need of decompression but are experiencing severe acute pain in the low back area, as well as for patients without any MRIs. In our office, however, we normally prefer to first have an MRI with candidates for decompression.

What is particularly special is that the VPADD's treatment is done with the patient in a standing position. The harness is placed around the patient's waist, and the upper torso is pulled to a point where the patient's heels begin to elevate off the floor. Once the patient is at this point, the chiropractor sits in front of the patient and proceeds to pull the pelvis in a series of motions, from extension into side bends, to encourage the disc to be reabsorbed or "sucked" back into place. Interestingly enough, patients who were not responding to standard decompression experience breakthroughs and diminished pain when trying this interactive procedure. We favor the VPADD's vertical approach, as there is less probability of irritating the area.

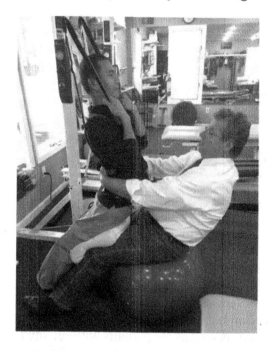

All the contraindications that were mentioned previously about spinal decompression still apply, though there is almost never any traction reaction with the VPADD.

You may find it difficult to find this procedure since it was developed here at the Back Pain Center. We encourage patients to share this information with their chiropractors with the hope of making this procedure more standard.

Chapter 8

The REPEX

In addition to spinal decompression, there are a number of other new or newly evolved technologies available today that can be of great benefit to healing your back. That's not to say that the examples in this or the subsequent chapters are the limit to treatments out there today, but we have found these to work well. In fact, I'd go so far as to say that when considering a particular chiropractor for a possible low back disc disorder, you might ask if he or she uses any or all of these.

The technology I'm describing in this chapter is a recent technological advance called the REPEX, developed by Robin McKenzie. REPEX stands for Repeated End Range Passive Exercise. Its original purpose was to offer patients with disc disorders an ability to do extended periods of prone press-ups, or lumbar extension, without having to use their own muscles. It employs what is called Continuous Passive Motion (CPM), which helps get motion and circulation into the low back area while also pumping out some toxins. It helps the patient regain flexibility and movement through extension without straining muscles, particularly in the cases where the patient may be too old to perform these movements on their own or is unable to do them sufficiently to make any difference.

The ability to set the table to different degrees of extension, along with its motor-controlled speed, has been an extreme help in patients with acute back pain who, due to their pain level, only have the ability to extend (bend backwards) one or two degrees. These types of patients are placed on the table while very slowly increasing the degree of extension so that, in 30 to 40 minutes, the patient will have increased their extension at least 12 to 14 degrees – a substantial change in patients who are safeguarding due to pain.

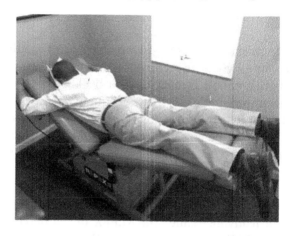

We have found the table particularly effective for patients with acute back pain who are locked or unable to move very much in any direction. The REPEX table uses a motor to bend the table at the waistline – just one degree at a time. That one-degree shift can be greatly slowed so it would take a full minute to complete one cycle. You can hardly see the table move! By slowly increasing the degrees and the speed with many of these patients, we can substantially increase the motion in their back in just one visit, up to twenty degrees in most cases.

Besides being an excellent tool for introducing extension to patients who are blocked from bending backwards due to disc herniation, we also use it very successfully with the sacroiliac upslip disorder. We have the patient lie on their side and hold the legs in place to create a stretch while the table bends approximately ten degrees. The table bends in the opposite direction of how is shown in the picture above, meaning that the center of the table comes up – this assists in gliding the SI back into place. The following video demonstrates this procedure.

https://youtu.be/4a2eust3pVU

I also find the table's ability to provide Continuous Passive Motion particularly helpful with seniors who have a significant amount of spinal stenosis and are in acute pain. We place these patients on the REPEX facing upward, knees bent with a wedge beneath them, and apply up to 100 cycles of motion to the low back area – meaning the table's CPM movement would repeat 100 times (again, with no muscle usage or strain on the patient's part). This does not cure their condition, but it can give them symptomatic relief that lasts days to even weeks.

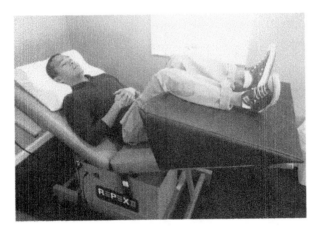

Doctors be aware: if you decide to try to regain some extension in a patient with spinal stenosis, be patient and only add one or two degrees at a time. If they feel any tension or stress as the table puts them into extension, even if it is just one or two degrees, you may hear about it tomorrow.

As an educated patient – be aware of this as well, so you don't find yourself getting in trouble. Be your own best advocate!

Also remember that you need to decide on a reasonable limit of time to allow for results before you proactively consider trying something else or trying another practitioner. Again, the key here is the educated patient. You decide, "I'm not going to jump to surgery. If this isn't working, let me try another office with decompression or simply another office that specializes in low back care." Then, give them a reasonable window of time to show results too.

Chapter 9
Laser Therapy

When it comes to elbows, carpel tunnel syndrome (hand and wrist pain), epicondylitis (tennis elbow), Achilles tendonitis (pain in Achilles tendon on the back of the ankle), knee pain, or plantar fasciitis (pain on the bottom of the foot), the laser can be truly miraculous and, in fact, can be the primary form of care. When it comes to low back pain, disc disorders, and sacroiliac issues, the laser is a complementary form of care used simply as an aid in the acceleration of patient recovery.

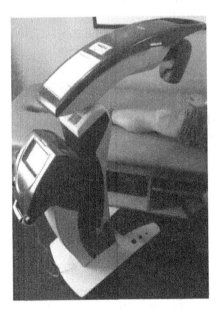

Rather than the types of lasers dramatized in movies or used by surgeons and dentists to cut tissue, we use a *cold laser* – also known as Low-Level Laser Therapy, or LLLT. It cannot cut or burn the patient at all, no matter how long it might be applied. There are also different types of cold lasers. In our office, we employ a class four laser, which is the strongest cold laser available. Ours is manufactured in Italy and is actually a robotic model, meaning we can set it for precise use on a patient. It also has two different frequencies, as it's been shown that one frequency helps reduce inflammation and stiffness, while the other reduces pain. Collectively, both frequencies accelerate healing.

How can it speed up healing? The laser light stimulates a part of the inner cells, called the *chromophore*. Stimulating the *chromophore* allows the injured cell to absorb oxygen and nutrients more efficiently and reproduce faster, which accelerates the ability to heal the damaged tissue, whether it's collagen or cartilage in joints, or ligaments and tendons. The laser also increases blood flow to the injured area, further allowing the cells to heal faster.

The benefits of laser therapy are even evident today for many patients with diabetic ulcers, whose wounds do not heal without the aid of laser therapy. Although laser therapy in the field of medicine has been around for years, it is still in its infancy. We will see that as time goes on, lasers will play a larger role in all branches of healthcare.

As wonderful as lasers can be in healing, I do not feel that they are sufficient as the only form of treatment for patients with low back pain. There are back care offices that really sell themselves as laser centers, but in my opinion – having probably the strongest and most advanced laser on the market – I find lasers to be a valuable adjunct to low back care, but not a chief player. However, in the other areas I previously mentioned (such as carpel tunnel or Achilles tendonitis), lasers really can be an effective primary therapy. We know this firsthand in our office, because even though we specialize in low back pain, about 40 percent of our patients come in for these, and similar, conditions.

Chapter 10
Electro Therapy And Ultrasound

Electric stimulation and ultrasound have actually been around for many years. Like laser therapy, I would also call these complementary to the more essential back therapies, such as spinal decompression, manual therapies, muscle energy techniques, and therapeutic exercises.

With electric stimulation, also known as electric muscle stimulation (EMS), electric pads are placed on the skin. These create tiny electrical impulses that feel like a tingling sensation but cause contractions in the muscles on which they are placed. This stimulation can be set to different frequencies and for different durations to encourage blood circulation to the region in order to promote healing, as well as to create different muscle reactions – ranging from fatiguing a muscle to strengthening it.

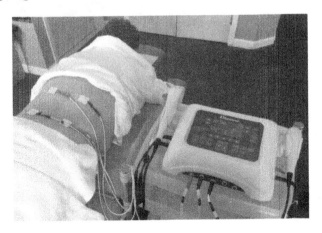

On the other hand, I have found ultrasound to be of greater assistance than most of the electric stimulation therapies. By ultrasound I do not mean the type used to see a baby in the womb; that is classified as diagnostic ultrasound. The ultrasound employed in therapy is therapeutic ultrasound. When used at a twenty percent output, it is an effective therapy to reduce inflammation in a joint. The sound waves penetrate six to eight centimeters deep to help disperse any excess fluid in the area (which is part of inflammation), while also helping promote additional blood flow to the area, all of which results in faster and more effective healing.

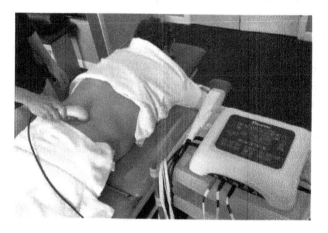

While surgery is necessary in certain cases, I would say the need is far less than the number of surgeries actually performed. Any patient with low back problems today really owes it to themselves to find someone who can provide effective treatment and hopefully turn their life around before resorting to surgery.

Chapter 11
Sitting: Hazardous To Your Health

Before I describe exercises that will benefit your particular issue, I first want to address some of the common activities that can cause or aggravate back problems. You will quickly note that these have become frequent everyday behaviors in our society – which is in part why back problems are such an epidemic today.

Plus, and this is very important – even if you are getting excellent treatment from a highly skilled provider, you won't improve if you are continuing bad habits that worsen your back condition. This is critical for you to realize. I have had patients whose treatments were not as effective as I knew they should be, only to discover that some activity or action by the patient was continuing to exacerbate the problem. Only after I brought attention to it and they altered this part of their lifestyle did we see great improvement.

I am certain this is the case for many people getting professional help. They think they are not receiving good care, when in fact they are countering all the positive effects of treatment by continuing the kinds of behaviors that either caused or worsened their condition. People with back pain too often begin programs with a healthcare professional only to give up when they see little progress, needlessly choosing to "live with" the discomfort or limitations.

In this chapter I will address one of the biggest culprits behind the unbridled frequency of back pain today. Learning what kind of patient you are (flexion, extension, SI joint dysfunction, etc.) to determine the right approach for you and following the perfect program won't necessarily help you if it is followed by poor sitting, walking, and exercise postures. Even these have *much more* effect on our lives than most of us realize.

We All Do It – All The Time

It's interesting how people will casually ask how we spent our day. We might answer by describing particular aspects of our jobs, a favorite form of leisure, studies, or other activities. But the true answer for the majority of us is that we spend most of our time: sitting.

Let's face it – we sit for breakfast, we sit in our car to drive to work where we sit for 40 plus hours a week, then sit as we drive home, sit as we eat dinner, and sit again as we watch TV or use the computer.

In fact, *think about how seldom we're not sitting.* Not often at all, except during sleep.

Unfortunately, coupled with most people doing less physically demanding activities and jobs, we've become a nation content to be sitters. In fact, there's a funny, and telling story where a chauffeur brings a new child to school as the teacher happens to be watching. The chauffeur opens the back door, picks up the child, carries him into the classroom and places him in his chair. Concerned that she wasn't notified about this problem, the teacher calls the child's mother to say, "I was never informed that your son, Johnny, couldn't walk." To which the mother replies, "Well, he can. But thank God he doesn't have to."

Oddly enough, I remember driving to school 40 years ago and hearing a news report on the radio that predicted in the next 30 to 40 years, the average work week would be between 20 to 25 hours, allowing people much more leisure time. They couldn't have been more wrong! I have patients working 50 to 70 hours a week. But I can predict that if this and other trends continue to dominate our activities, we will only see *more* back problems.

Why? Because sitting may be the single most hazardous activity you can do for your back. Most of us never think about it, which is perhaps why we are doing it so poorly.

Sitting Is Simply Hard On Our Bodies

One of the biggest problems with sitting is lack of motion. You are not moving – your body isn't moving. But the body is *designed* to move.

You take motion away from any particular area and it starts to suffer. We're sitting so much that our joints and organs are stagnant for long periods of time, so now our circulation isn't moving as it should be, and neither is our lymphatic system. A Consumer Reports study on health in the February 2012 edition cites research has found that even amongst people who exercise every day, long periods of sitting can increase their chances of getting cancer. With extended sitting, we are reducing the motion that allows muscles to continue pumping, a process by which toxins are expelled, so I can understand that being so dormant could contribute to causing cancer.

Australian researchers have also noted that prolonged sitting is linked to increases in key biomarkers, including inflammation, insulin resistance, and waist circumference. In contrast, interrupting long periods of sitting with even one or two minute breaks each hour has been found to lower these body markers.

Improper Sitting Creates Sacroiliac Joint Dysfunction

Adding to the inherent problem of sitting too much is sitting improperly. Most of us don't pay much attention to *how* we are sitting. We don't think it is significant and take it for granted; until things start to hurt and we can't figure out why.

Among other things, sitting "incorrectly" puts a significant amount of stress on the sacroiliac joint. This is critical to appreciate because once the SI joint is misaligned and out of proper position, the entire foundation of the spine becomes compromised. This creates abnormal pressure on the soft tissues surrounding the vertebrae such as ligaments, tendons – and the discs.

While I might advise most everyone to get more physical activity and exercise into their daily schedule, the reality is that our lives today *will* involve a lot of sitting. So how can we do it better? How can we sit so that we are *supporting* our bodies rather than stressing them?

Proper Sitting Posture: Starting With The Basics

Let's start by creating a good supportive posture, especially at work. Be sure not to cross your legs or ankles, and make sure your ears are lined up above your shoulders and that your shoulders are lined up above your hips.

Additionally, if you are using a computer, it's important to position the screen so that it is at the height of your face. What do I mean by that? Try this: sit at your desk, close your eyes, and sit tall. Now open your eyes – your nose should be pointing to the center of the computer screen. If it is not, get creative and put some books under the screen or do whatever will help position it correctly. You can also find monitor risers and laptop stands specifically designed to raise the screen to the proper level.

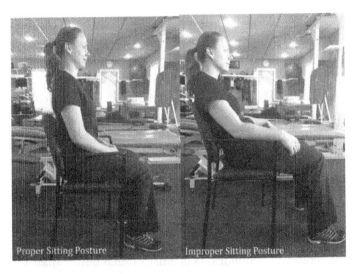

Proper Sitting Posture   Improper Sitting Posture

A side note about reading at the computer or just sitting to read: many of us get to a point where our eyes need some assistance. We go to the local drug store and buy "off the rack" ten-dollar reading glasses. I would advise that you visit an optometrist and get prescription glasses specifically designed for reading, and particularly for computer use (which would have anti-reflective coatings and a focal distance about 20 inches, among other things) since we spend so much time at the computer.

Beyond the kinds of glasses we get, many of us will wear them at the end of our nose and peer over the top when we are not reading. This will eventually cause neck and back pain, with radiation down into the arms. This actually happened to me. As I began feeling pain radiate down my arm, it dawned on me that my posture was causing the problem. I went out and purchased progressive lenses – with the upper part of the lens being clear – this way, I didn't have to look over the top of the reading glasses when I was talking to patients. In a very short time, my arm was fine.

Regardless of the circumstances, if your head is tilted forward, it can aggravate a back condition and interfere with low back recovery.

Low Back And Leg Positions

I've seen patients purchase chairs literally up in the thousand-dollar range. However, regardless of their cost or quality, if you do not sit properly, they won't be of any help. To be honest, I have not found any particular chair at any price that will serve as a panacea. What I'd suggest is to simply find a good chair with good support where you can put a McKenzie lumbar roll behind your back (provided you are not stenotic), which can be found on the Internet for about twenty-five dollars. This works much better than buying a thousand-dollar chair. You can buy a firm or medium roll – whatever suits you best – and position it exactly where it fits you best.

If you are an extension type patient, it is especially important to have a lumbar roll if you are experiencing pain resulting from a disc disorder. Be sure to slide your bottom as far back in the chair as possible, and once your bottom is positioned, bend forward and place the roll as shown: just above the belt line.

Yes, there are some patients for whom a chair's built-in lumbar roll works well – but not usually as well as they may think. This is also true for patients with luxury cars whose seats have built-in lumbar support. I generally tell them to turn off the car's lumbar support and buy the twenty-five dollar lumbar roll.

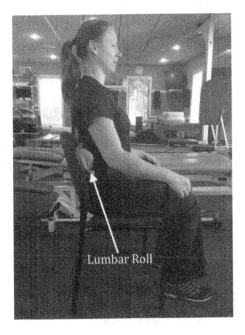

Lumbar Roll

Whichever chair you choose, be sure that it has a good back support and that your chair's height allows you to have *both feet flat* on the floor. This is very important. Even many inexpensive office chairs have hydraulic lifts in their shafts that allow you to adjust the height. The general rule for chair height is that it should allow your thighs to be horizontal to the floor with your feet flat on the floor.

Now, if you are very short or very tall, you may have a challenge. If you are short, you may need to place a footstool, a box, or other object under your feet to raise them so that your thighs will be at the desired horizontal position. You definitely don't want your feet hanging off the edge of the chair.

If you are very tall, you may have to elevate your desk and even use a high bar stool type of chair to accommodate your height to allow your thighs to be horizontal. The more your knees rise above your hips, the more that intradiscal pressure increases.

Now let me *fine-tune* this for you.

Extension type patients may be okay if their thighs are slanting downward, the knee being lower than the hip area. Flexion type patients who are in pain may want to increase the height of the knees so the thighs are slanting upwards, with the knees higher than the hips. Flexion patients must understand that although this may bring relief, it isn't ideal and is a compromise to normal body mechanics. If you begin to feel relief, try to gradually readjust to where your thighs are horizontal. Plus, if you can get to a point where you are able to do "posting" (explained later in this chapter), then you are heading into a more optimum state, back-wise.

Especially For SI Patients

For patients with SI joint disorders, there is a way to sit that will help relieve the pain caused by the pressure placed onto the ischia, or sitting bones. I have found that sitting on a contour pillow with the larger portion of the contour under your thighs, while simultaneously incorporating the McKenzie lumbar roll, will reduce the amount of abnormal pressure on the SI joints.

Sitting on the contour pillow if you are a combination of SI and extension, or SI and flexion, should not be a problem. The only difference would be that the extension type must incorporate the lumbar roll, whereas the flexion type should not.

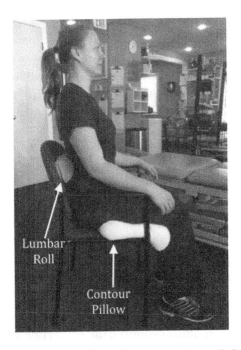

Lumbar Roll

Contour Pillow

Additionally, an SI patient can do an exercise while seated in this position. On the side where they feel the pressure and pain, they press down on the knee like they are trying to push their foot into the ground, while at the same time "lifting" the leg against the pressure of their hands. This is an isometric exercise – nothing is actually moving – but it will help relieve some of the pain in the SI. They should do that on both sides, but always start on the painful side.

They can also do what is called "seated bicycling." Starting in the same seated position, they push the left knee forward and pull the right knee back, then do the reverse – the right knee forward and the left knee back. This is all performed while the feet stay flat on the floor (or footstool). They would do between five and ten of these every hour.

Proactive Sitting: Posting

As I said earlier, part of the problem with sitting is the lack of motion. Yet, even while sitting, we can do small movements to increase the motion in our back and body, in addition to the exercises I've already mentioned.

"Posting" can be done while sitting and is very effective in bringing relief and increasing low back mobilization and circulation. It is similar to posting while on horseback – if you have any familiarity with riding horses – where a rider "bobs" up and down in the saddle in rhythm with their horse's trotting gait.

Depending on whether you are an extension type patient or a flexion type patient, posting will need to be tweaked as shown in the video below. Extension type patients should sit straight up and move the belly button forward – rolling the pelvis forward. It helps reinforce the correction of the disc tissue.

https://youtu.be/LQ7QCpBxuNs

On the other hand, if you are a flexion type patient, you want to move the belly button forward slightly, and then move it backwards as far as you can while sitting properly. The difference is that you are trying to move the belly button forward in an attempt to regain some of the extension abilities, provided it does not increase pain, but roll backwards to provide immediate relief. This should be done with a slow but steady gradient. Reminder: the extension patient should not add the backward motion.

There is a slight variation on posting done for the SI patient. They should use their abdominal muscle to pull the belly button inward (essentially tightening the core) at the same time as rolling the pelvis backward.

Do note that even if you are using a McKenzie lumbar roll and you find it helpful, don't assume that there is no need for posting. There is only one thing that will give you the benefits of motion, and that's motion.

Diaphragmatic Breathing

We breathe all the time, 24 hours a day. It's something we've done since the day we were born. Yet as adults, most of us do it incorrectly.

Think of it this way: the diaphragm is to the body as a conductor is to an orchestra. It affects our whole system far beyond what most of us realize. Again, this is part of the miracle of the human body – one that needs to be understood and appreciated.

Most people use the diaphragm improperly. When you breathe in, your abdominal or belly button should move outward. When you breathe out, your belly button should move inward. Not only is this relaxing and overall healthy for the body's organs since it was designed to work this way, but it also helps mobilize the low back with gentle and slight flexion and extension motions.

Most of us weren't taught to breathe this way. When I ask my patients to show me how they breathe, they breathe in and the shoulders go up and the upper chest expands. Yet, the two key muscles in the body that were designed to work 24/7 are the heart and the diaphragm, not the shoulders, trapezius muscles, or chest muscles. Besides it being physiologically wrong and altering the biorhythms in the body, it can only lead to tension and stress in the shoulder area due to overusing muscles in a way for which they were not designed.

https://youtu.be/5GtuejbRsNk

Practice breathing how I've recommended in the video above. Make it a part of your everyday routine. When you are doing diaphragmatic breathing while sitting, you should feel a little motion in your low back. Again, that subtle motion is so beneficial to the body.

Timing Is Everything

Again, I am intentionally spending a considerable amount of focus on improving your sitting, and so should you.

A good tip to help you ingrain good posture, and to do your posting or isometric exercise while sitting at work, is to buy a relatively inexpensive watch timer or set your phone to alert you (on vibrate if ringing would be a problem in your workplace) every 60 minutes. This will serve as a prompt for you to reflect on how you've been sitting over the last hour. If you find that you are slouching, then correct the posture and do some posting or other appropriate movements if there is pain.

Another Tool For The Extension Patient

In addition to the lumbar roll, there is a tool, called the Nada-Chair, made particularly for the extension type patient. It has been on the market at least as long as I have been in practice, yet I am surprised at how few chiropractors and physical therapists are aware of it. It is truly a wonderful device, though admittedly a bit strange looking and many patients have refused to wear it mostly out of embarrassment.

The Nada-Chair is a device worn around the back and over both knees. When you tighten the straps, it forces you to maintain an extension posture.

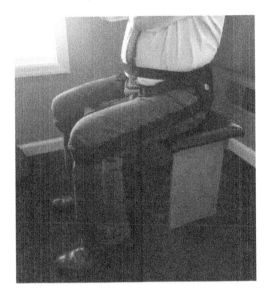

If you're "bold" enough to give it a try, be sure to periodically loosen the straps and do the posting exercises. The Nada-Chair can also be found online at www.nadachair.com. The cost is around 70 dollars.

Sitting has obviously been around since we began walking. It has probably always been an issue regarding back health, but has only more recently become a *major* issue due to how much we sit today. Yet there's another current, relatively new issue causing immense problems to our back health for people of all ages – of which most of us have no idea.

Chapter 12
Texting: Growing Pains Of The Tech Revolution

Texting. It's pervasive. People of all ages communicate this way, far more than talking on the phone, or talking face-to-face. This significant change in our culture has arrived with hurricane force, and is forever altering how we relate to each other.

It is also changing how we relate to our back.

Don't be fooled: this innocent activity may produce the most dramatic shift in spinal problems over the next 10 to 20 years. While it is too soon to know yet, my strong sense is that we are going to see more back problems and surgeries than ever before. The harm caused by texting goes far beyond injuries sustained from poor lifting, sports, or mowing the lawn. It's much bigger, as texting is already a consuming activity for millions every single day.

It is estimated that heads are slumping over smartphone screens on average from two to four hours daily. Doing so creates a very unnatural posture, with a person's neck severely bent forward for long periods of time.

Let's keep in mind that the typical head of an adult weighs from 10 to 12 pounds. Yet, there will be *many times* this amount of pressure on your cervical vertebrae when you bend the neck at such a steep angle – it's estimated that each inch that the head is bowed forward causes an additional ten pounds of stress on the cervical spine and shoulders. This constant forward flexing radically burdens the neck.

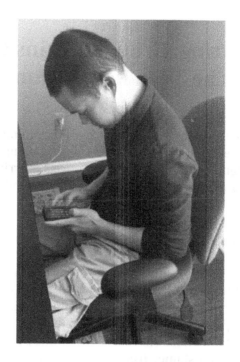

The reason we emphasize good posture – be it while sitting or standing or during most any activity – is that it lowers the stress on all areas of the spine. It's how we were designed to be. When we violate this, especially with regularity, we're setting up structural problems not only for the spine, but also for issues affecting the nerves and what they control, creating all kinds of mechanical and neurological issues. Plus, problems in the cervical spine will usually translate into compensatory problems in the low back as well.

This imminent epidemic of new issues should serve as a warning to everyone – particularly to parents. Many people won't feel the ill-effects immediately as it will be cumulative over time (averaging perhaps 60 to 120 hours per month based on the daily two to four hour estimates!). It can weaken neck and back muscles along with connective tissues and discs, until the only remedy may be surgery.

In fact, research already shows that college students are reporting neck pain as a result of texting, with many also suffering shoulder pain if they text even more frequently. This new development may well be the equivalent to our recognizing the damage done by people sitting at computers at work for eight hours a day, their typing leading not only to back and neck pain, but also carpel tunnel syndrome, tendonitis, and other problems. The damage from ongoing texting may be additionally compounded by frequent long periods of searching the Internet, watching YouTube, and playing games on their phones, as well as staring down at tablets, e-readers, and other mobile devices.

Parents need to realize that this is not a minor issue. We are hearing of children experiencing pain as a result of texting as young as three years of age! This could be one of the most dramatic shifts we've seen in structural problems on our younger generation. While I'm putting emphasis on children regarding this issue, make no mistake – it will affect everyone. In fact, adults may feel its effects sooner than kids, even though they typically don't put in as many hours texting.

Certainly texting is here to stay (until some new technological development replaces it), so the best you can do is reduce the amount of it, while also improving your posture while texting. Hold the phone (or tablet or other device) up to your eye level. Plus, take regular breaks every 15 minutes or so. Obviously, exercise and having good posture habits in other areas of your life will help, too.

Chapter 13

Backpacks Lead To Back Trouble

The use of backpacks is different from texting in that it is not nearly as consistent or universal. However, the use of backpacks has increased exponentially for students of all ages, from elementary school through college, as a means to carry textbooks as well as other items, including laptops for older students. By the time students are in high school, they may be carrying 25 to 30 pounds, especially as some feel that they don't have time to go to their lockers between classes and so carry all their books for the day.

When I was growing up, at least posture was discussed in school. Now, it isn't addressed at all. Yet, wearing a backpack for school actually educates the body to stoop forward, creating potentially lifelong poor posture. In fact, the weight and size of backpacks are doing more to create future back patients than any single activity after texting and sitting.

How it affects each child will be different, particularly at different ages. It can certainly be said that children of elementary school age don't have the strength to keep a correct upright posture while carrying these heavy loads, putting their skeletal systems under significant stress. When placed on the shoulders, the backpack's weight can pull a child backward. To compensate, the child will likely bend forward at the hips or arch the back, which can cause the spine to compress unnaturally. This will cause kids to develop shoulder, neck, and back pain, as carrying these heavy backpacks can create rounding of the shoulders, strained muscles, and even irritation to the joints of the spine and rib cage. Furthermore, it can alter the middle and low backs' natural curves. This can all lead to immediate problems or ones that will surface after many years.

Plus, many backpacks have taut, thin straps that burrow into shoulders and can hinder circulation and possibly nerve function, leading to numbness, tingling, or weakening of arms and hands. Even worse, many students, either out of convenience or because it looks cool, will carry their backpacks over one shoulder. This will stress the muscles even further as they try to compensate for the unbalanced load, their spine leaning in the opposing direction. This strains the back and ribs greater on one side, potentially leading to muscle spasms and pain.

As you evaluate the situation for your own child, consider if he or she has begun complaining of back pain or numbness/tingling in his or her arms or hands? Do you see them bending forward or sideways, trying to compensate for the heavy backpack? How can you help limit this risk that seems to permeate today's culture for your own child?

Fortunately, there ARE numerous things you can do:

- Weigh the backpack and lighten the load. It is suggested that students do not carry more than ten percent of their body weight in a backpack, according to the American Chiropractic Association (ACA)
- The backpack should have two wide and padded adjustable shoulder straps to balance the weight on the shoulders. Teach the student to adjust the straps so the backpack rests close to the body rather than sagging toward the buttocks
- A waist belt can help diminish the burden on the shoulders as it places some of the weight bearing onto the waist/hips. While students might be

reluctant to use the belt between classes, they
certainly could take advantage of them for longer
walks to and from school

- Pack textbooks and heavier objects at the bottom
center of the backpack, low and close to the body,
while avoiding having sharp objects near the back
- Multiple compartments can better help students
disperse weight of the contents in the backpack
- Teach the student how to lift properly, bending at
their knees and not the back as they use both
hands to pick up the backpack and place it onto
their shoulders
- Advise the student to leave books in their locker
as much as possible during the school day rather
than hauling the whole day's books around
- Suggest they only take home those books they
need for studying that night. Or even better – get
a second set of textbooks at home so your student
doesn't need to bring them home every evening.
Even though this may require extra expense on
your part (many textbooks are available for
purchase online), it may be far cheaper than the
medical expenses resulting from injuries

You can also get a backpack on wheels, however, be aware
that these tend to be heavier overall and possibly harder to
bring up stairs or roll through snow. Also check with the
school before purchasing these rolling backpacks as some
schools won't allow them due to the potential for tripping
other students in school halls.

Simple Ergonomic Solution

While all of the above suggestions are good, there is also a simple solution for kids to improve their posture: wear their backpacks on the front. The result will be a generation of kids that will be standing a lot taller and have significantly less back problems in the future. The video below shows the difference between how wearing a backpack on the back slumps the student forward, while a backpack worn in front helps improve posture.

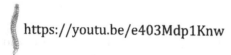 https://youtu.be/e403Mdp1Knw

I'm sure it would not take much for manufacturers to tweak the present design and make it specifically front-fitting, but until they do, your student can wear the one they already have in this manner. If your child is too "embarrassed" to wear it in front at school until the practice becomes more commonplace, then perhaps it could at least be worn this way when walking home. (I should point out that we haven't done any studies regarding the safety factors when wearing packs in front as far as falling or tripping, so we can't unreservedly recommend this, but know that overall this would be a better approach for posture.)

It appears that the use of backpacks by students is here to stay for the foreseeable future, so the best we can do is to determine how to avoid causing further problems for our children or ourselves.

Let's continue exploring how to minimize back problems and their accompanying pain, by instead of looking at what we put *on* our bodies, to examining what we put *inside* our bodies.

Chapter 14
Problem Diets Contribute
To Problem Backs

Contrary to what some believe, being overweight may not be the cause of your back pain. There are as many patients with back pain who are thin as there are those who are overweight. This is by no means an invitation for back pain sufferers to be heavy, as many other health conditions can accompany being significantly overweight. But as far as diet and back pain, weight may not be the cause – with the exception of spinal stenosis and degenerative joint disease.

However, much of what we eat does cause an *inflammatory reaction* in our bodies. Sugars, white flour, sometimes dairy, and many processed foods will create inflammation in our tissues that can interfere with the ability of our tendons, ligaments, and muscles to recover and function at their best. So what should we do?

There are hundreds of diets jockeying for the title of being the best. Unfortunately, we have been taught to think that there is some magic bullet – a new enzyme or vitamin – that will compensate for all of our bad eating habits and give us that desired state of health. I personally once went to a doctor in New York City who had me taking 80 vitamin and mineral pills per day.

I'm not saying that vitamins are useless or completely ineffective, but that you simply need to be a bit more cautious. If you have a problem, then educate yourself and realize that there's more involved than simply going to the health food store and asking the salesperson, "What's good for high blood pressure? Or colitis?"

Either you or a professional should do some research. If you seek a professional's help – be they chiropractors, nutritionists, physician, etc. – find out their philosophy towards vitamins. Be aware that even many nutritionists use vitamins and minerals the same way allopathic doctors use drugs.

Basically, allopathic medicine will use drugs to create the opposite effect of your symptoms. If you have a fever, you take something to bring the fever down. If your blood pressure is high, you take medications to lower it. I'm not criticizing this as good or bad, as it may be necessary in certain conditions, but it has little to do with trying to bring the body back to a healthier state by correcting the cause of the problem. Unfortunately, many in the health field have jumped onto this same bandwagon and promote vitamins and minerals as the "solution" for a particular problem. My suggestion is to find a professional that will try to balance body systems instead.

Additionally, you can't eat unhealthy food and expect vitamins to make up for your deficiencies. I know some people contend that foods today are deprived of the vitamins that they used to contain due to different farming methods. But there are stores, like Whole Foods, that have high quality organic and healthy versions of basic foods. You might consider it a luxury to purchase such foods, though you'd also save the cost of sodas, cookies, and other junk food. Besides, what is your health worth? How expensive is it to correct medical problems that might otherwise have never manifested if you ate really well?

We Really Are What We Eat

Our bodies are essentially self-contained, waterproof units. Except for the air we breathe, the liquids we drink, and the foods we eat – not much else comes in. So naturally, what we breathe, drink, and eat will have a profound effect on our body. It's really a compliment to our bodies that we can take in so many toxins and chemicals in our air, water, and especially food, and continue to function relatively well.

The simple thing about diet is that it's not so much what to eat – but more about what *not* to eat. The probability we will discipline ourselves not only to find the right diet, but also to implement all the many do's and don'ts of that particular diet is, in most cases, not going to happen. And in reality, it's not necessary.

If you want to lose weight, increase your energy, feel more mentally alert, be more optimistic, have regular bowel movements, and increase your probability of living a longer, healthier life, then start applying the Dr. G (that's me) common sense rules regarding dieting.

> ➤ Eat foods as close to their natural state as possible
> ➤ Stay away from sugars and flour products
> ➤ Don't mix too many food groups together in one meal
> ➤ Start the day with 16 ounces or more of water, at least 30 minutes prior to eating
> ➤ Don't drink large quantities of water while eating
> ➤ Try not to eat past 6:00 PM
> ➤ Less food is really better

Let's take a moment to examine each of these rules.

As you can see, my number one rule about food is that the further you move away from a food's natural state – especially toward today's plethora of processed foods and snacks – the greater probability that it's not good for you. I'd also include processed meats here, as there are too many steps between their original state and when you eat them.

Knowing all of this can make many decisions pretty simple and straightforward. Let's look at the other suggestions.

> Stay away from sugars and flour products

The second rule is to stop eating products made with sugar and/or white flour. Not only are these two products bad for your health, they cause an inflammatory reaction throughout the body, which will exacerbate pain and delay the proper healing time. Sugar and white flour will age you prematurely, interfere with your blood sugar levels, elevate cholesterol, produce anxiety, and interfere with sleep. Those are just a few examples, but they should be enough.

I'd particularly stay away from soda – a sure killer. Depending on the brand, you'll get anywhere from eight to eleven teaspoons of sugar from one can alone! That is way more than most candy bars, yet some people drink soda all day long. You should also know that another skyrocketing disease today is diabetes. In fact, we are beginning to see adult onset diabetes *in children*, all as a result of our obsession with sugar-loaded products and flour-rich fast foods.

> Don't mix too many food groups together in one meal

We have come a long way from man's early ancestors, and although intellectually we have changed a great deal, physiologically we have not. Eating food from different parts of the planet in one sitting would have been impossible a thousand years ago. Yet today, in one sitting, we can eat fish from Norway fried in corn oils, foods from the Midwest, nuts from Hawaii, and oranges from Florida. The digestive system is not designed to perform these multiple types of digestion simultaneously.

Why is this important? Think about your digestive system. We eat a big steak and potatoes, and finish with some fruit and/or a sweet dessert. Common sense tells us that meat takes hours to digest, whereas fruit takes a significantly shorter time and are assimilated much quicker. Eating fruits or desserts at the end of a meal will cause those foods to sit in the digestive tract substantially longer, making them become either putrefied or rancid – not a pleasant thought.

> Start the day with 16 ounces or more of water, at least 30 minutes prior to eating

Water is critical to our well being. People are often amazed when they read that our bodies are made up of about 70 percent water. That should be a clue right there! But most people today suffer from some level of dehydration. Some of that is due to substituting sodas and coffee for good plain water, but much of it is also simply due to not drinking enough water throughout the day.

To that end, I suggest first getting into a simple habit of drinking about 16 ounces of water as soon as you awaken. Your body gets dehydrated overnight and needs to be replenished right away. Doing so may also alleviate much of the sluggishness many feel in the morning.

Become more aware of how much water you drink throughout the day, and know that thirst is not always a good indicator of how much we need. It is recommended that we drink eight to ten glasses of water per day. To some of you, that may sound like a lot. But if you make a conscious effort, you will find that your body will get used to it – even *crave* it – as you give it what it needs. In fact, sometimes when you're feeling tired or not thinking clearly, just drink a glass or two of water and see if that doesn't perk you up and make your mind sharp again.

➤ Don't drink large quantities of water while eating

The irony is that one of the rare times when you should *not* drink a lot of water is when you're eating. Drinking large amounts of water during your meal will dilute the digestive enzymes that help break down food, interfering with their ability to get those precious vitamins, minerals, essential fatty acids, carbohydrates, and proteins needed for good health.

➤ Try not to eat past 6:00 PM

You'll note that I suggest trying not to eat late at night. Eating later not only contributes to greater weight gain, but it can also interfere with vital sleep as your body is still working hard digesting instead of relaxing so it can fall into a deep, restful sleep.

I realize that eating earlier can be difficult as people now work more and come home later. Unfortunately, these longer workdays tend to have us eating less nutritious meals as we choose the simple ease of fast or prepared foods. One way to combat this is to plan meals in advance. Planning basic, healthy meals ahead of time can help prevent last minute decisions like ordering pizza and a liter bottle of coke. Some people even pre-cook meals – a day ahead or longer and freeze them to later heat up and serve.

➤ Less food is really better

In our society, malnutrition is more a function of *what* we eat rather than not eating enough overall. We can eat plenty of food and still be malnourished, as is becoming increasingly evident. People today are much more often overweight and obese rather than too thin.

Better choices and less food overall is really the suggestion here. As far as food and diet, I would recommend the book *Edibolic Stress – How the Lies You Are Being Fed Are Making You Sick!*, by Dr. Michael Rothman, as a good source of information. As I've said, you really need to research in terms of what and how many vitamins to take. That is also true with the foods you should eat. Dr. Rothman's book is a good start.

More About Water

Increasing water intake is something I really push with my patients. Sometimes I'll ask them, "Do you drink much water?"

"Of course. I have two cups of coffee in the morning, a ginger ale in the afternoon, and fruit juice with dinner."

"And where's the *water*?" I'll inquire.

"Well Doc, all these products have water in them."

Many patients think of fluid as synonymous with water. It isn't. Let's take ginger ale, for instance. They do start with water. They add some artificial coloring, some artificial chemical flavoring, and six to eight teaspoons of sugar – and there you have ginger ale. Yes, there is water in it, but how many steps removed from its good natural state? Don't think for a second that drinking soda, coffee, or beer has the same effect on the body as drinking good clean water.

Unfortunately, tap water should be avoided as it contains toxins, such as lye and fluorides, along with many other chemicals. You can filter your water or purchase spring water that is significantly better than water from the tap.

With regards to water, there are actually different opinions on *how* to drink it. Some nutritionists recommend sipping small amounts of water throughout the day. It is my belief that you will hydrate the body better by drinking large amounts of water – sixteen ounces at a time – four to five times throughout the day. Sipping small amounts throughout the day is like giving your grass a quick sprinkling – the water never gets deep enough to hydrate the bottom roots. The same is true with the body.

Small amounts of water never get to the secondary areas of priority. If there is an inadequate amount of water, the brain and the digestive system will get it first. This can cause a problem for many other areas of the body, and certainly does when it comes to backs, as the discs are supposed to have a high percentage of fluid. On MRIs, we frequently see that vertebral discs are often dehydrated (which can be determined by the vertical thickness of the disc, and the coloration or shading one sees on an MRI).

Now, if the water intake is low *and* there's also a lack of mobility, discs will deteriorate at a significantly higher rate than normal. That deterioration is basically due to the poor vascular supply in discs; discs depend on motion to aid in the transport of fluids in and out of the tissue. Low fluid intake plus lack of mobility accelerates disc degeneration in anyone's back.

I'd advise that drinking adequate amounts of good quality water is a key factor in anyone's back care and general well being. To that end, I've already suggested getting into the habit of drinking about 16 ounces of water upon waking up, since your body gets dehydrated overnight. But don't make this water part of your breakfast. Instead, drink some good quality water early on, well before you eat. Do your morning back exercises, take a shower, and brush your teeth, so as to give that water time to move through your system before you start your breakfast. Remember that drinking large amounts of water while eating will only dilute the digestive enzymes that help break down food and absorb needed nutrients. This is a basic change you can implement right away that could make a big difference in your overall health.

Healthy Life

I would venture to say that *very* few of us have any idea how great we could feel if we had very healthy diets, complemented by sufficient exercise, intake of water, and sleep. I think it would be extraordinary! The human body *is* truly amazing. If you do the right things for it – without looking for the "magic bullet" to solve all your problems – you'll be surprised how quickly the body can respond. But a word of warning: as remarkable as the body is, it can get to a point where it can't turn around if a health problem exists.

So, don't put off living a healthier life – start now.

Chapter 15
Drugs And Surgery: When You Need Them

One area in which I may differ from many of my colleagues is with the use of medications in handling low back pain. You will hear arguments that pain is the "warning signal from our bodies that something is wrong, so why would you want to hide the warning signals from the person?"

Although there is validity in that argument, not taking medications or waiting too long to take medications *can* create more of a problem than originally existed. In fact, there are as many patients who stay on medications much too long as there are patients who wait too long to start. All too frequently, when patients are asked if they take medications, they answer, "Only when it hurts," or "No doc, I don't want to mask the symptoms."

Now, if you are at home dealing with your back problem without any medical help, then perhaps this approach to tough it out may not be such a bad idea, since covering up a problem (with medications) and doing nothing to correct it could cause you to do more harm. In that regard, using the warning signal of pain as a barometer for your back problem isn't a bad idea. Because here is the caution: taking medications like Advil, Motrin, or other over-the-counter non-steroidal anti-inflammatory drugs (NSAIDs) when things start to hurt can cause you to put off seeing a DC, PT, or MD that specializes in low back pain. This will allow the condition to worsen, possibly causing more damage and requiring more assistance to remedy. It's important to differentiate the aches of daily living from true nerve pain caused by a mechanical problem that needs care.

For instance, taking two Advils before a round of golf is, in many cases, a good idea if you are sure your body aches from golf are due to arthritis (though that doesn't mean you can't improve your condition with proper help). So take the Advil. But recognize that even in such cases, or any point where you need some type of NSAIDs, be sure you are on the *appropriate* exercise program to help you strengthen and maintain a healthy back. Also, be aware of any *change* in patterns. That is, if you would normally feel achy around the 15th hole but notice that you're now consistently getting pain sooner, realize your back issue may be progressing. You may need to increase your exercise protocol or, even better, get a professional to examine you. Simply taking more Advil is not the solution. *It is important to understand that what's fixable today may not be fixable tomorrow.* Waiting too long to get help is equivalent to letting a simple cavity turn into an abscess.

Do know that there isn't a book – even this one – that will ever take the place of a professional who truly understands how to evaluate and treat back disorders. Please do not avoid seeing the appropriate professional who could significantly help your condition.

If your condition is not worsening and you choose to "tough it out" without medications, be sure to read the descriptions in chapter 17 to determine which exercise protocol is appropriate for your pattern. Give the exercises two or three days. If you start to improve: great. On the other hand, if you do not see a change or you seem to be getting worse, then seek help and don't be afraid to take any prescribed medications. Most patients are off the medications in a relatively short time.

Taking NSAIDs

If you decide it is time to incorporate over-the-counter medications, take them as prescribed on the box. The one exception to this is: depending on your size, you may need to increase the quantity. Advil, for instance, recommends taking 200 mg, or one pill, every four to six hours. The directions are the same whether you are a 95-pound female or a 250-pound male – the instructions don't take your size into account. But you should *always* ask your physician beforehand if it would be appropriate to increase the dosage. Realize that taking four Advil may be equivalent to taking a prescription dosage.

If approved by your physician, take the NSAIDs. My suggestion is to take them for a five-day program. Adhere to the box's instructions as to how often to take them. If it instructs to take the medication every four hours – then do so. Continue taking the anti-inflammatories for five days, even if your pain diminishes, while you incorporate the proper exercises. If you notice an improvement at the end on the five-day program, you can start to cut down on the NSAIDs while continuing to incorporate the exercises and proper body mechanics in terms of sitting, standing, driving, laying down, having sex, and so on.

Please note that I'm not suggesting you go on this five-day NSAIDs program if you have just developed a mild backache. It's more appropriate in situations where your back issue isn't easing up and is becoming a recurring problem.

Seeking Professional Help

If after incorporating NSAIDs you are still having trouble, even with the exercises, then you need to seek help. Inform the treating DC, PT, or MD which medications you have tried, along with the exercises you have been incorporating and your experiences with them.

Medrol Dosepak

Once the DC, PT, or MD that specializes in the treatment of low back pain evaluates you and it is determined that you were correct in the choice of exercise protocol, he or she may recommend or put you on a stronger prescription anti-inflammatory, along with a proper treatment plan. These medications are not meant to be taken for an extended period of time. If you see little or no improvement, you may be taken to the next rung in the ladder and given a *Medrol* Dosepak. This is a steroid-based anti-inflammatory and is significantly stronger than NSAIDs. If you have reached this level of care and treatment, an MRI should be ordered as well to better determine your condition.

In terms of the *Medrol* Dosepak, most doctors give this as a six-day program where you will take 6 pills on day one, 5 pills on day two, 4 pills on day three, 3 pills on day four, 2 pills on day five, and 1 pill on day six. With more severe low back conditions, particularly those related to disc disorders, we have found that incorporating two *Medrol* Dosepaks at the same time works best, provided your prescribing physician approves. Therefore, take 6 pills on day one, open the second pack and take another 6 pills on day two, take 5 pills on day three, and then 5 on day four; continue with this pattern until day twelve. Again, please consult with your physician before doing so.

Depending on the severity of your condition, it may be the decision of your treating doctor to bypass the Medrol Dosepak and going directly to an epidural.

Epidurals

If after taking the Medrol Dosepak while being compliant with the therapy and home care you are still not progressing, the next step would be to see an anesthesiologist for a consult to determine if you need an epidural. By this point, if you are still in pain and showing little change, an MRI must certainly be ordered if it hasn't already. I believe most professionals wait too long before incorporating epidurals, as they can be a valuable part of treatment and recovery.

Epidurals are done in surgical centers, with the patient partially or completely sedated as a steroid is injected into the spinal cord area. There is now an even more advanced procedure called a *trans-foraminal epidural,* which appears to be more effective and specific than regular epidurals.

An epidural powerfully reduces inflammation to allow the back to get better and heal. I'll give an analogy, while not very elegant, that gets the concept across. Imagine a cat has gotten its head stuck in a chain linked fence and can't get it out. The anti-inflammatory would decrease the swelling in its head and the therapy would then be able to pull the head out of the fence. By the same token, the epidural will help make your therapy protocol more effective, and so assist in your improvement long after the epidural wears off.

It should be noted that chiropractic and/or therapy centers that do not have a relationship with an anesthesiologist might find that the anesthesiologist will order the patient to suspend therapy during the two-week period following an epidural. This, in my opinion, is a big mistake. Yet, I have been in situations where the patient was told "no therapy" while I'm telling them that this is the exact time for therapy. In reality, there is no reason for this caution against therapy, other than what we're seeing more and more in the healthcare field that is sometimes called CYA, or "cover your ass." Anesthesiologists – not knowing the therapy office to which a patient is returning – would not risk that a treating DC or PT would irritate the problem only to have the patient find fault in the epidural.

In reality, the two to three weeks following an epidural or *trans-foraminal epidural* is the most critical time to get therapy. In our center, the anesthesiologists to whom we refer for *trans-foraminal epidurals* insist the patient continues with therapy immediately following the injection. Instead of simply being a narcotic to help deal with pain levels, epidurals are a type of medication that complements treatment dramatically.

Surgery

There are three key scenarios in which waiting and "toughing it out" may be counterproductive and surgery might be the appropriate action.

One is if there is a significant loss of strength in the lower extremity, particularly if the foot has "dropped" due to weak muscles. Another is if a significant atrophy is noted in the lower extremity, such as a shrinking of the leg. The third is if there is any loss of control with bladder function as a result of the back problem.

Otherwise, if the pain can be tolerated and you persist with home exercises and good ergonomics in your daily activities, you most likely *will* get better. Fortunately, we only have a handful of patients that ever reach a point in care in which we need to decide between surgery versus slowly moving forward with therapy.

This degree of success is a result of several things: the knowledge gained over time by specializing in low back pain, the patient following specific and appropriate exercises, and the incorporation of new healing technologies. We can improve backs without surgery better than ever before. The old adage that "time heals all wounds" has a lot of merit in regard to backs. The patient that can truly persist on a quest to get better and stick to their specific exercise program can find "miracles" do happen.

Chapter 16
Judging Results

Change, no matter how small, should occur relatively soon in the professional treatment protocol. If you, the patient, are now into your tenth or twentieth treatment without changes to your condition, then perhaps the treating doctor's treatment plan might be questionable.

The dilemma for all patients getting any kind of therapy, not just for the back, is that they have no reference point as to the doctor or therapist's capacity to get results. It's different than going to a restaurant and knowing after one visit whether we're going back, because we can reference our experiences from all other restaurants in which we've eaten.

That's not so with healthcare. How do you know if the doctor you're seeing is doing the best job for you? Hopefully this chapter will give you insight as to results you can rightfully expect.

Setting A Reasonable Time Frame

A reasonable window of time within which you should see improvement will vary based on your condition. If you have had symptoms of severe spinal stenosis for about two to three years, you will have to be patient and be very aware of the *subtle* improvements that indicate you're actually getting better. In fact, some patients with severe spinal stenosis should realize that preventing the condition from getting worse might be their best option.

However, if you have had low back pain for only three weeks, I would say that somewhere within three to five visits you should be able to say "Hey, I think I see improvement or a change here." If not, is your doctor investigating further and changing his or her treatment plan? Is the doctor looking to see if there may be another, better approach?

Everyone is an individual and, therefore, each back condition is individual. However, there are a reasonable number of visits within which you could expect to see some improvement – not necessarily a cure, but at least improvement. If you're told that it will be four months before you feel any improvement, *that* could be a red flag and something to reconsider. Four months may be fine before *correction* happens, but when it comes to feeling some *relief* – that should be much shorter than the time needed to correct the problem.

Therefore, I think it's a good idea to ask the doctor before treatment commences, "How much time before I can expect to see improvement? Would it be unreasonable to expect improvement in three visits? Five visits?"

We recently had a patient with pain down his leg. After an evaluation, we did what we call a hip-hike, which is a very gentle way of putting the SI joint back into position. It's a corrective exercise that's actually done by the patient. The patient then got up and walked down the hall to see how he felt.

"Man, I'm really impressed! That sign really means what it says."

He was talking about the sign outside our office: "Same Day Relief Care."

Improvement Isn't Always All Or Nothing

The truth is, there was still some pain down his leg, but it had been greatly diminished. There were still more treatments to be done, but I bring up this example – and mention our sign – because getting at least *some* relief from pain should not have to take very long.

If your doctor is on the right track, you should generally begin to see results within a two-week period, depending on the degree of severity. Improvement can be judged not only by how you feel, but also if you've seen any improvement in function. Are you able to walk a little further? Are you sleeping better? Is your energy improving?

A mistake some patients fall into is the "all or nothing" law. They either feel completely better or, in their viewpoint, the care isn't working at all. Always talk to your chiropractor about your progress. If you are treated and on the next night you notice an improvement in your sleep pattern – even if it only happens for the first night and then goes back to square one by the time you return to your treating doctor – let them know you had a good first night. *That feedback is vital.*

In all fairness, the more your treatment protocol is in the direction of the flexion type patient, the longer progress will take and the more gradual it will be. If you are a flexion type patient, the goal is either to stop your condition from getting worse, or to try to slowly and gradually increase your ability to extend. For patients with severe spinal stenosis, a very difficult diagnosis to treat, you may only see a five percent improvement within that first two- to four-week period of treatment. Again, hopefully your chiropractor can give you a realistic expectation for your condition.

Combination Approach

Lastly, back pain is sometimes not necessarily a one-profession solution. This is where I believe patients and professionals need to become more aware. When asked, many patients who have not improved with care will tell you that they tried chiropractic...they tried physical therapy...they saw an orthopedist...they have even had epidurals.

One would think that this patient has tried it all, yet there is one thing they haven't tried: combining multiple therapies. Often times, combining chiropractic and physical therapy (PT) together achieves better results than either could alone. In many cases, if chiropractic and/or PT didn't work, adding an anti-inflammatory during care can turn results around. If the patient is still not improving, then we look at going to the next stronger medication, which could be prednisone. If that doesn't work, we look at adding an epidural along with therapy (as described in chapter 15). I can't tell you how many patients turned the corner only after incorporating complementary therapies at the same time. For that reason, you may want someone who is open to complementing their own work with that of others to achieve the desired results.

Never Give Up

The point is this: just because you tried some – or even many – protocols does not mean you can't be helped. Case in point, I recently had the pleasure of treating a new patient, Pam, who had suffered with low back pain for 15 years. Pam is a 45-year-old with average body weight who tries to be active by going to the gym and working hard at attempting to feel better. But her pain caused a significant degree of interference in normal day-to-day activities, and overall, was something she seldom could forget. Pam was told that she had severe disc degeneration in her low back area and that after years of physical therapy and chiropractic therapy, she might have to live with the pain. I treated Pam and after the second visit, she was and has been completely pain free.

It was telling to see Pam's bittersweet reaction to the results we obtained. As ecstatic as she was, Pam was also very angry about the years of suffering she felt that she had needlessly endured. It's totally understandable, and the reason I encourage you to find the treatment that works for you.

Do not give up. Not all practitioners or protocols are the same, just as no two patients are the same. The human body is a remarkable healing machine – I've seen this time and time again.

Correction After Relief

While your first goal may be to feel better, you ultimately want more than just relief from pain. You don't just want to get to the point where you're out of pain and then stop treatment – you want to correct the problem so it doesn't happen again. You want an improvement program that will help heal the issue, while also building flexibility and strength to prevent re-injury.

So again, how can you know if you're actually getting better and should continue with a program to *correct* the issue? The biggest clue that you're on the right track toward correcting the problem is that you should continue feeling *relief* along the way. If your condition is getting better, you should also be *feeling* better, or at least seeing functional improvement. For example, if you've lived with pain going down your leg for three months and in three weeks it is gone, I would think the doctor is on the right track and that continuing to work with them for correction is something you want to do.

I would define a corrective treatment program as more of a program to strengthen and stabilize your back – to reinforce the correction and reduce the probability of any reoccurrence. The ultimate goal is to pass the ball over to the patient by teaching them exercises they can do at home on their own, free of having to get chiropractic care or with a significant reduction in chiropractic care (perhaps down to once a month).

The Right Kind Of Doctor

I truly encourage co-creating a reasonable plan with your chiropractor for when you should begin to see results. That way, you can properly judge whether or not you're getting the right treatment.

This is especially true when it comes to the treatment of low back pain, as there are many different beliefs of its causes and, therefore, approaches to treating it. Some doctors will tell you it all starts from the feet up, while others say it starts from the head and neck down. There is even an MD in the New York area that insists almost all back pain is emotionally caused. Now, I believe that low back pain can be partially caused or worsened by emotional stress. But to claim that almost all back pain is emotional in nature and requires psychotherapy that could take two to three years is, in my opinion, irresponsible.

There are also doctors who respond to a patient not improving by *blaming it on the patient* – that the patient must be doing something wrong and that it's never the doctor's fault. This is not the doctor you want.

I'm not saying that I have all the pieces to the puzzle when it comes to back pain. But after over 35 years in practice, and after dedicating over 20 years specifically to the treatment of low back pain, I can tell you that I have many of the pieces. A big difference is that I know when I *don't* know. That is, I stopped insisting many years ago on having to be right. I know when we aren't getting the results I would like and therefore should try a different protocol, or even try to work with another discipline in tandem with my treatment plan.

I hope to inspire you to find the right doctor *for you* – even if you've tried some before without results. As you are learning from this book, some approaches are better for different patients. Hopefully, by being armed with more knowledge, you will better understand your situation, when to continue staying under a particular chiropractor's care, or when it is time to pack it in and try someone else.

You want a doctor who will outline your treatment plan, tell you when you can reasonably expect to both feel better and correct the issue, and one who is open to shifting treatment plans if you are not seeing results within those time frames. Insisting upon these is your responsibility. After all, it is your body. Who else should advocate for it?

Chapter 17
Sacroiliac, Extension, And Flexion Pattern Exercises

I would have to presume that most of you reading this book have been dealing with back pain for more than just a brief period. However, if you find yourself experiencing a severe flare-up as part of ongoing issues with your back, and it's just too unbearable to do anything, then bed rest may initially be necessary to get some relief.

If after reading chapter 5 describing different types of back pain patterns you see that you fit into the flexion category, then in all probability lying on your back with a pillow under your knees will be the most comfortable position (but you likely knew that already from experience).

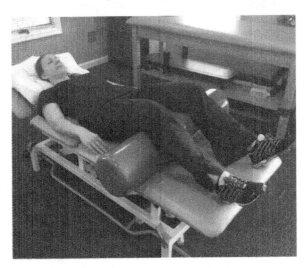

On the other hand, if you are an extension type patient, it is useful to know that you have a greater likelihood of experiencing a sudden acute onset of severe or extreme pain. In your case, lying on your side with the painful side up and a large pillow between the knees should help significantly.

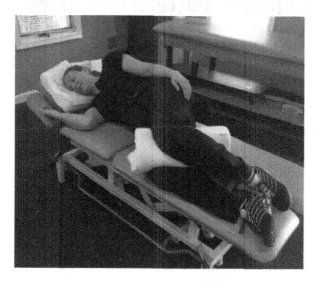

However, bed rest alone is usually not sufficient to truly get you out of pain. There are specific exercises you can do on your own that will better bring you relief, as I will explain in this chapter.

Your Program At Home

In describing the exercises that get you out of acute pain, I will suggest trying a specific movement. If that exercise is too painful, then you should shift to a more basic variation of the movement that you can do comfortably. These more basic movements I will detail as well.

I'll be presenting some of these exercises on a gradient – starting with the ideal exercise to perform for your condition, and then moving "downward" to simpler alternatives. That is, exercise "A" is preferable. But if you cannot do "A", then try exercise "B", which is a little easier. If you cannot do "B", then try "C", or even "D". If you can do "D" – stay with it a little – then try "C" again. It should be a little easier this time. The goal is to ascend back up: as you stay with "C" successfully, move up to try "B" again, and eventually "A". Each time you get to the point of, "Oh, I can do that one," then continue to move up the scale of exercises.

Doing small amounts of these exercises more frequently throughout the day is better than doing large amounts just once or twice, so you may end up doing these exercise patterns four to six times a day.

Ice And Heat

Before giving you the exercises, I want to emphasize that using ice on your back is excellent during these acute cycles. Many people go right to heating pads as they are convenient and seemingly give initial relief. Icing in the acute flare-up will actually provide more relief and help.

Why? First, understand that when there is irritation to a nerve or joint, there's inflammation. Heat will make things *expand*, but you already have an area where the nerves are inflamed or expanded. You're trying to put the fire out. Ice will do this much better. Ice application acts as a natural anti-inflammatory, whereas heat will actually increase circulation to an area and worsen the issue.

In fact, the commonly suggested protocol of staying with ice for the first twenty-four hours after a low back injury and then moving on to using heat is simply not true. There's no legitimacy to this at all. You *stay* with ice on your low back when it's a joint-nerve problem. The only exception is if you are a flexion-type patient with a lot of degeneration, achy muscles and tightness – then heat may work better. Otherwise, for the SI and the extension patient – ice works significantly better than heat.

What is true for *everyone* is to only ice for 15 minutes at a time. That's because after 15 minutes of use, the effects of ice *reverse*. Ice reduces inflammation by taking blood out of the area. But the body can only take so much blood away from the area. Eventually, the circulation needs to come back in. So at the end of 15 minutes, it is important to stop icing and take a break. If you were in an acute condition and wanted to be very aggressive with ice, then use it for 15 minutes once every hour.

So, what is the best way to apply ice to the back?

If you feel okay lying with your back on the floor, put your legs on a chair seat to create a little bridge and slide the ice beneath you. That will press the ice against the back, which is preferred. If that's a painful position and the only position offering relief is resting on your side, then you will somehow need to prop the ice against your back while on your side. I recommend going to a pharmacy and purchasing a relatively inexpensive elastic low back support. Strap the ice against your back with the belt around you to help the cold penetrate deeper.

Now, even though I call it "ice," I really prefer freezable gel packs, especially those made for injuries. Many of them are flexible – that is, they don't get too hard – and also don't get too cold, but that's largely a function of your freezer's temperature. Even if the gel packs come out rigid, most will soften up in a few minutes and mold to your back. Most commercially available packs are only 6 x 6 in size. In our office we offer 12 x 14 gel packs that cover the entire low

112

back and fit really well into back belts, so I recommend purchasing one of the larger gel packs.

Now, once you're able to get out of bed, it is a good idea to strap the ice against your back using the belt again and walk around a bit. In fact, most of the time when a patient finishes therapy in our office, we put ice on their back with an elastic lumbar support and have them walk on the treadmill for 10 to 15 minutes.

Trust Your Body

Let me give you another important, yet seldom addressed, ingredient in healing a back: *you need to trust your body.*

I've seen patients who have become so fearful of injuring themselves further that their whole lives revolve around not experiencing pain. That is a big mistake. They are so afraid of having another back attack that they're cautious in everything they do. But once you start to get better, you really need to trust your body. Yes, you could hurt yourself again, but in most cases, the body is not as delicate as it seems to people with back conditions. You don't want to sacrifice the experience of life to get through all your days in a pain-free state.

You can start to depend on your body again, as long as you sit properly and follow the guidelines outlined in chapter 18 to make your daily activities supportive of your condition. Once you are better, you don't have to do a fifteen or thirty-minute exercise program to remain healthy. Eventually, you want to get to a point where you do a two- to five-minute morning routine. Doing basic back exercises and applying the suggestions in this book on proper posture while sitting and driving allows most people to return to nearly every activity, from golf to skiing to running (provided they do those things properly as well). These activities are available to most people with back problems, no matter how severe.

Getting Out Of Bed

Now, some of the exercises can be done while in bed, while others are better served if you do them on the floor. So first, let's address the simple act of getting out of bed.

If you are at such an acute stage that you need to be in bed for the day – so be it. But it is important that you make an attempt to get up and walk. I will go into further detail about getting out of bed in the next chapter, but I wanted to include it here since you may be getting out of bed to perform some of these exercises.

Remember, always roll to your side and use your hand to push yourself into a seated position, making sure to engage (or squeeze tight) your abdominal muscles while coming up. Be sure to exit on the side of the bed that allows you to come up with the painful side up – meaning, if your low back pain radiates into your right leg, you want to get out on the side of the bed where you can roll onto your left side and then get up. You can also see a demonstration by accessing the following video.

https://youtu.be/YISSzAGTfC0

If you find that getting up is painful, you might look again at the chapter on medications to see what you can take to allow for some activity. Do note that even if it is painful to get up, there will not be any damage from the attempt of getting out of bed. In most cases, patients are more cautious than necessary. But be realistic: if getting up is just too severe, then give yourself some additional bed rest.

Now let's look at the exercise program for you. Do note that although we've tried to categorize exercises into three different categories, there will be exercises that overlap.

Sacroiliac Exercise Program

It is important to realize that with all of these exercise programs, you are not doing exercises that will cause any permanent damage. Most pain you might experience (if any), especially any sudden spasms, is a defense mechanism from the body.

The only criteria for not starting with the sacroiliac program is if it is too painful to lie on your back, or if you get more radiating pain into your extremities as you attempt the exercise. Remember, if you are experiencing any weakness in the lower extremity or a significant amount of atrophy (shrinking) of the leg in the lower extremity, seek professional help immediately.

Accessing the video links shown here will be very helpful to see exactly how to do these exercises.

A. Hip Hike

Let's assume you are an extension patient with a bit of a sacroiliac condition. If you are not able to get on your back due to pain, skip this for now and go directly to the extension protocols in the next section of this chapter – the prone press-up.

On the other hand, if you are an extension and SI type patient and *you are okay on your back*, let's try to perform a hip hike.

Let's start with the side with the most pain. If the pain is centered in the middle of your back, then you can simply choose on which side to start. If you feel an increase in pain during the performance of the hip hike, then switch sides and see if the other side is less painful. If it is, start with that side and do five to ten reps. Try the painful side again and if you can, do five to ten reps on that side as well.

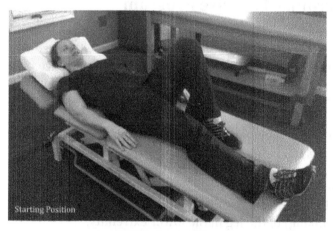

Starting Position

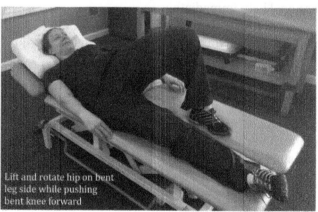

Lift and rotate hip on bent leg side while pushing bent knee forward

B. If the hip hike is too difficult or too painful when trying to lift and rotate, place a towel or your hands around the knee on the painful side and pull that knee toward your chest. Push moderately against the resistance of the towel or hands. Repeat this exercise on each side three to five times.

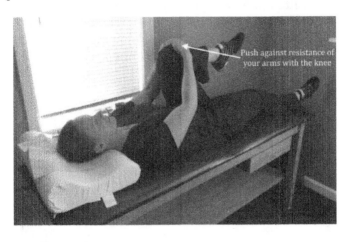

Push against resistance of your arms with the knee

C. If pulling the knee is simply too painful, then bend the knee on the painful side with the foot flat on the floor, keep the other leg straight on the floor, and perform five to ten crunches by bringing your nose to your knee. Note: do not do full sit-ups.

D. If you are unable to do crunches, simply press down on the floor with the foot of the bent leg. Do this five to ten times.

Depending on the level of pain, challenge yourself to try the next gradient of difficulty – that could mean the same day, the next day, or even next week. This next video will demonstrate the hip hike, as well as its modifications.

https://youtu.be/cn2PF5dEW8g

A. Prone Press-Up (Or Cobra)

If you find that you are comfortable *lying on your stomach*, then let's attempt to do a prone press-up (or cobra). Begin with your hands under your shoulders. Then, press up with the use of your arms only – your back muscles should not be involved in try to come up into the cobra position. Slowly lower yourself.

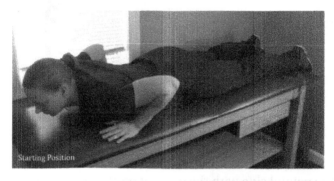

Starting Position

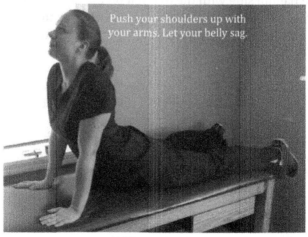

Push your shoulders up with your arms. Let your belly sag.

B. Realize that you may not be able to do a full prone press-up, or cobra, at first like you may have seen in yoga postures. So, begin with your arms under your shoulders, lift up just two to five inches using your arms, and slowly lower yourself. Repeat this activity five to ten times, or more if you keep seeing improvement. You will see that as you continue to perform this activity, your ability to come up higher will increase – this is a productive sign.

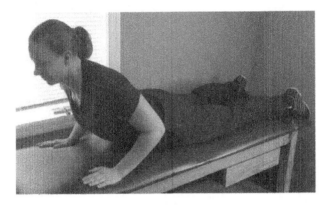

C. If that's too difficult, go to a lesser gradient and try to lift just your head and shoulders off the floor. The following video will show you the prone press-up and its modifications.

https://youtu.be/LkA35oYimkw

For those of you who skipped to this section, once you've gotten past the acute pain stage with the help of the prone press-up exercise, now you can try the hip hike.

Butterfly Crunch

Once you've completed prone press-ups and hip hikes, try to do a "butterfly crunch." Lie on your back with knees bent and pointing outwards on the floor with the bottoms of your feet together.

119

Note that a "crunch" is *not* a traditional full sit-up. You are not bringing your body up and forward like a sit-up, but rather a pulse upward like you are bringing your nose straight towards the ceiling. Do this exercise 10 to 15 times.

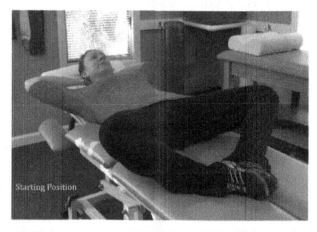

Starting Position

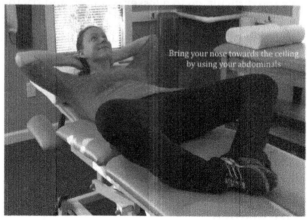

Bring your nose towards the ceiling by using your abdominals

If you have any concerns about neck pain, clasp your hands behind your head with your fingers interlaced to support it. If you can, create a pelvic tilt at the same time by rolling your pelvis up and backward. It's a great exercise to stabilize the SI joint.

Butterfly Bridge

The next exercise is a "butterfly bridge". While still on your back in the same position as a butterfly crunch, lift your hips off the ground.

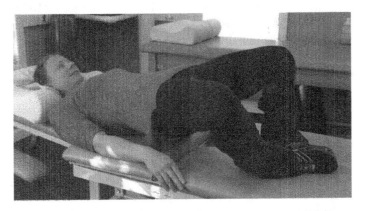

Pelvic Tilting

After the "butterfly bridge," get on your hands and knees if you can and slowly start pelvic tilting: pull your stomach in and round into a camel back while keeping your abdominals tight, then arch your back into extension, looking up at the ceiling and still keeping your abdominals tight.

https://youtu.be/Wb7PS3SflYM

Next, you will lie on your stomach and do ten prone press-ups again to a height with which you are comfortable. Then, turn over and finish with the very first hip hike exercise (or the variation that applied to you).

That's It!

That's your program! It's not that difficult and the whole routine is only about five minutes long. However, if your pain is not changing, repeat the program three times a day. Remember to strap a gel pack onto your back and take a walk after each round.

But again – realize that exercise and icing aren't going to help as well *if your ergonomics are wrong*. If you sit in a slouched position on the couch, it's not going to help you. *Maintaining the proper ergonomics and doing your exercises for the first three weeks is critical for things to begin to stabilize and heal.*

Unfortunately, I'm sure there are many patients (even some of my own) who have done the exercises diligently, but don't correct their ergonomics. Then, when they don't get better, they assume that the exercises don't help and stop doing them. I am presently treating a patient who actually did very well with the exercises, but continued to have residual leg pain. Everything else was fine, but he still had a little numbness on the side. He figured he was fast becoming a candidate for surgery.

But I said to him, "You know, Mike, when I look at you standing and sitting, your head is so far forward, it hardly seems like it's on your body."

He had no sense of what I was telling him. I had him stand up and showed him how to stand properly. He, like many people, thought that standing with good posture means to move their shoulders back. But I corrected, "No, don't push your shoulders back. All I want you to do is lift your sternum (your breast bone) up toward the ceiling as high as you can go while keeping everything else relaxed. That means don't lift your shoulders – that's also key. Your shoulders should be totally relaxed." When you stand like this, it's literally impossible to put your head in the wrong position.

So I asked how it felt with this posture. He said, "I feel stupid. I feel like people will laugh at me because I'm leaning backwards." I took a photograph while he was in this posture and he had to agree when I said, "You don't appear stupid at all. You look perfectly straight."

He was so unaccustomed to it, that it felt strange and unnatural. I instructed him to set his phone timer for every hour and to simply assess and correct his posture whenever it rings. After doing so for two to three weeks, the brain will be programmed to think about posture every sixty minutes.

Interestingly, by week two, his leg pain had disappeared even though we hadn't made any drastic changes to his protocol – just the act of checking and correcting his posture every sixty minutes. He was on his home exercise program *and* paying attention to ergonomics. That subtle action of bringing his head back two inches was enough to take pressure off the nerve.

The beautiful thing about good posture is that you don't have to be focused on it 24/7. There are certain things in life that you have to stay focused on all the time. Climbing a mountain isn't a time when you want to let your mind wander. But with posture, as long as you check it periodically and correct it, you will get the benefit. If you catch yourself three to four times a day and lift up your sternum, or "breast bone high" as we say in my office, you'll see improvement!

The Extension Exercise Program

The pure extension patient is one with a disc herniation and radiation down the leg. The exercise program is very simple:

the key exercise is the prone press-up, or cobra. You do small amounts repeated until you are feeling well enough to turn over and add the SI program, because the prone press-up alone does not stabilize or strengthen the core. That's what the SI program does. So, no matter how comprehensive your extension program, you want to incorporate the SI program.

Fortunately, it won't hurt extension patients to do the SI exercises, which is why I presented those first. In fact, extension patients usually have a disc herniation coupled with an SI joint dysfunction. In most cases, doing the SI exercises is not contraindicated – it doesn't work against the extension type condition – so you should try the SI program first. But again, if you're in too much pain at first to do any of the SI exercises, continue doing the cobra in small amounts, 15 to 20 of them, with ice after. Remember, doing them frequently throughout the day is far better than one marathon session.

A prone press-up is a great exercise for a disc herniation. The goal is to get as far up as possible. Move up further *when you can* and you'll slowly see an increase in flexibility. It's okay if it's somewhat painful in the back, as long as the back pain stays localized. If you're doing the extension exercise and notice the pain traveling down your leg, then you need to back off. This is when you may want to return to being on your back and staying with the SI exercises.

https://youtu.be/LkA35oYimkw

Once you're able to fully get up in the cobra position, it is time to incorporate breathing. This is very simple. On the way up, breathe in. Then, stay up as you breathe out. As you breathe out, let your belly sag.

A big lesson to learn from this is that prone press-ups can and should centralize the pain, meaning the pain should localize to the point of origin and away from the extremities. That is, *you* can control your discs, not the other way around! So, keep repeating this exercise until you start to see the pain centralizing.

The Flexion Exercise Program

It should be acknowledged that the flexion program is actually a compromise. It's not ideal for healing the body mechanics. With a flexion patient, we have a person with a history of bad posture their whole life, and so the body has somehow adapted to it and the patient feels better in this bent-over position. Now, at the age of 68, they are developing back pain. They start walking and they're surprised to find that it is painful. It is the accumulation of years of poor posture, though some part of it may be genetic.

The first result we want for the flexion patient is relief. The "compromise" I referred to is that the flexion program is designed to make the person feel better, but not necessarily to improve their posture. But once they start to feel better, we are then able to work on improving some of their extension, or posture if possible. We want to *slowly* incorporate some posture protocol, because too much extension too quickly will flare up pain in the flexion patient.

Seated Toe Touch

Sit on the edge of a sturdy chair and lean forward to touch your toes. Hold for five to ten seconds, and then slowly come back to an upright position. Depending on the severity of your condition, do this three to ten times, one to three times a day.

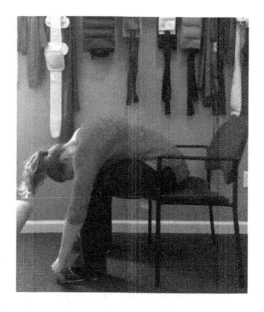

Knee To Chest

Lie on your back with both knees bent and feet flat on the floor. Bring one knee to your chest with the help of your arms and hold for five to ten seconds. Do the same on the other side and repeat the routine five to ten times.

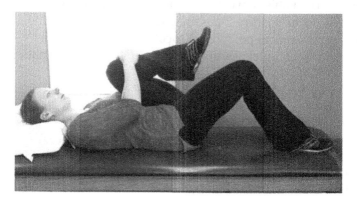

Knee To Chest With Crunch

This exercise is slightly more challenging than simply bringing the knee to the chest. Be mindful of your neck when doing this exercise – if elevating the head off the bed or floor produces pain, do not incorporate this exercise.

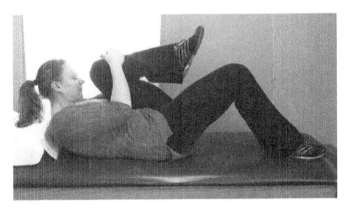

Once again, with the help of your arms, pull your knee to your chest and attempt to bring your nose in the direction of your knee. Do this on both sides, five to ten times.

Pelvic Tilting

This is another exercise performed while lying on your back with both knees bent and feet flat on the floor. In this exercise, you attempt to push your low back into the floor, which will naturally tilt your pelvis back. Hold for five seconds, and then relax. Repeat this five to ten times.

Pelvic Tilting With Crunch

You should also consider your neck with this crunch variation. If you feel any pain when elevating your head, please do not do this exercise.

While laying on your back, push your low back into the floor and gently elevate your shoulders two to three inches off the floor for a count of five seconds. Do this five to ten times.

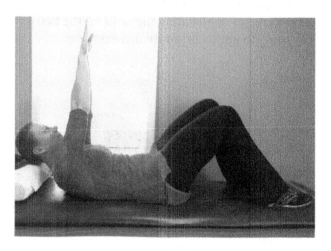

Bridge

In the same position as for the pelvic tilting, lift your pelvis up towards the ceiling and hold for five to ten seconds. Repeat this exercise five to ten times.

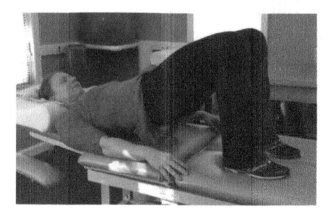

Single Leg Bridge

Again, this may be more challenging and if you sense any discomfort, do not force yourself to do this exercise. While lying on your back, keep one leg straight and only bend one knee. The straight leg does not have to be elevated, and I recommend you start with it on the floor or table. Lift your hip on the bent leg side two to three inches off the floor, hold five to ten seconds, and relax. Repeat this five to ten times on both sides.

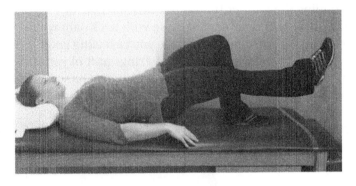

That's the flexion exercise program! Depending on the severity of the condition, you can do this routine one to three times a day. As I mentioned before, these exercises are designed to bring relief so that once you're better, you can slowly start to incorporate extension with the help of a professional. You can see these exercises in motion below.

https://youtu.be/8YtJA_UJ2HU

No Pain? – Then Stretch!

If you're not in any pain, or your pain has subsided from doing the exercises - do you still need to exercise at all?

Following the exercise protocols, including the cobra, is still a great morning program. The only other area to focus on would be stretching some key muscles. That is, once we relax or make the person feel better (and have them strengthening the core), there are some key traditional stretches they should do.

Most people don't realize that the one muscle group with the most profound effect on the low back is the hamstrings. If you had 100 people in back pain – and you weren't allowed to examine them other than check their hamstrings – you would find that 80 percent of those with back pain would have hamstring problems. So once you're feeling good enough, make stretching your hamstrings part of your daily protocol. Place your foot on top of a chair seat or some other object not too high off the floor, and while keeping that leg straight, move your chest forward while maintaining a vertical posture.

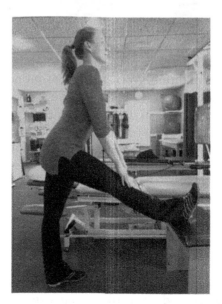

Remember never to "bounce" the stretch. Stretching any muscle is best done with slow, progressing movements. Stretch somewhat, hold it, and then stretch further if you can and continue this pattern. All stretches should be held for at least 30 seconds to be of any benefit.

By doing the exercises in this chapter that are appropriate for you, and maintaining good posture, many of you will be surprised to find your back pain diminish and the ability to perform many activities improve. However, how you carry out your normal daily activities will play a large role.

Chapter 18
Making Daily Activities Safer

The simple things we do daily will either help, hurt, or be neutral to our backs – from brushing our teeth, to putting on shoes, to eating breakfast, to walking to the train station, and so on. This chapter will describe how to at least make these activities neutral, and at times even beneficial.

While these recommendations are especially for people recovering from back pain, they can be applicable to everyone. They make life easier for your back, which may help keep you from incurring unexpected back injuries in the future. This should also serve as a wake-up call to people, especially as they get older. I hear from patients all too often, "Doc, I don't understand it. I used to do these things all the time without any problems!"

I have to explain that you can "get away with" a lot more when you're younger. But you're not the same person you were even ten years ago. Your body mechanics change. Mentally, we may be feeling like we're 20. We have a great youthful attitude, are excited about living, curious about the world, and eager to try new things. But the truth is, our bodies are just not going to do what they used to do 15, 20, or 30 years ago.

So, while it's great that you think of yourself as a young person, once you get over 40 you have to start thinking of your body more in terms of ligaments and tendons, rather than just building muscles and strength. A ligament is the tissue connecting bones or cartilage at a joint. A tendon connects muscle to the bone. You may have the muscular strength to lift weights, but your ligaments and tendons may not. I have many patients who don't want to give up weight lifting – particularly older men with big muscles. They're in a lot of pain, but the idea of losing their muscles is so upsetting to them that they won't stop lifting. They need to take on a different viewpoint of who they are. As do you.

The more you give your body what it *truly needs* – good flexibility, balance, posture, and nutrients to an area to cause the ligaments and tendons the least amount of inflammation – the more life becomes enjoyable and pain-free. We become more "extroverted" in how we live, which is much more fun. If you're in pain, your life becomes introverted; you're thinking about your aches. You begin to lose that simple joy and appreciate that you once had energy. That's *not* fun.

Besides realizing that who you were yesterday isn't the same as who you are today, you should also know that what's fixable today may not be tomorrow. It's possible that the ground you lose by not sticking to a good back program may not be regained. You need to understand the seriousness of maintaining what you have.

The focus in this chapter is to provide recommendations for normal daily activities in order to live a life as pain-free as possible. Remember, there can be variations on how to do these actions depending on whether you're in the extension category, flexion category, or sacroiliac category.

Getting Out Of Bed

Here is a critical factor that can affect your entire day right from the start. Don't just jump out of bed in the morning if you're getting over a back problem.

If you're an extension type patient – you may especially feel achy in the morning, since mornings are typically the worst for you. That's because after having taken all the weight off your feet for a number of hours, your body has had little gravitational pressure on it and the discs tend to fill up with more fluid than usual, so *any* disc problem becomes a little more exaggerated in the morning. Know that this is normal if you are an extension type patient. Before you get out of bed, lie on your stomach and elevate your shoulders slightly by getting up on your elbows. Do this a number of times. If you can, gently go higher. The higher you go, the better prognosis for a good day.

When you're done putting some motion back in your back (I often tell patients that it's like putting oil into a gate hinge), then roll to the side of the bed with your painful side up – that is, if you have low back pain that radiates down your right leg, you want to be on the side of the bed where your left side is down before you get up. Then, you come up sideways by using your arm to push off the bed until you are upright. You may need to switch which side of the bed you sleep on since you want to get up sideways with your pain side upwards. What you *don't* want to do is hook your hand under your hip and perform a sit up to get out of bed. That is pretty detrimental to a back patient.

Now, if you're a flexion patient – you generally feel pretty good in the morning. You may want to roll onto your back and rock with your legs bent into your chest so as to loosen up and get some motion into your back. Just as with the extension type patient, the flexion patient should never just sit up. They should roll onto their side and get up sideways as well.

From Sitting To Standing

Let's follow through the next step. You're sitting on the edge of the bed and ready to stand. First thing to do is slide your bottom to the edge of the bed, tighten up your abdominal muscles, and come straight up by pushing against the floor with your feet. Once you are up, it's a good idea to walk around with tall posture for a minute – sternum high towards the ceiling, shoulders down and relaxed.

A side note especially for older patients or seniors: once you stand up at the edge of the bed, you should not take your first steps immediately. Sometimes it takes a few seconds for the circulation to adjust from lying down to standing. If you were to stand up and instantly take a few steps, you may find that by step two or three away from the bed, you get lightheaded and fall. Instead, once you stand, stay in that position briefly. If you start to get lightheaded, then plop right back down to sitting on the bed. This approach is strongly suggested to avoid risk of falling and fracturing a hip. Fractured hips are one of the leading causes of death in seniors. Here is the video again on how to properly get out of bed and transition from sitting to standing.

https://youtu.be/YISSzAGTfC0

Once you're up and able to move, it's a good idea to walk around – get some motion in your body. It would also be a good time to dedicate the next five minutes to your home exercise program, regardless of whether you're an extension or flexion patient.

In respect to doing exercises, I would also suggest you apply a similar consciousness about getting off the floor after doing exercises. Getting off the floor should be very calculated until it becomes second nature. While on the floor, roll to your side, get on all fours, place one foot forward, and come straight up while trying to keep the back as vertical as possible. If you are feeling unstable, have a chair or other stable object beside you to assist you in getting up.

Brushing Your Teeth

The simple act of brushing one's teeth has sent more people to The Back Pain Center than one can imagine!

If you are an extension type patient, lean into the vanity and maintain a slight arch in the low back area. You may need to place a towel around you since it's not the neatest way to brush teeth, but washing a few extra towels is well worth preventing another back episode. I personally put a foot up on the vanity and stretch my hamstrings while I brush. But this should *only* be considered if you are sure your balance isn't a problem and you're feeling pretty secure about your back.

Now, if you're a flexion type patient, you could lean over and place your body weight on the vanity with your elbow or hand, and do pelvic tilting or posting. Flexion patients have lost a significant amount of mobility in the lumbar spine and any opportunity to regain this motion should be used to their advantage.

Taking A Shower

Extension patients may need to bring in a stool or other object on which they can place a foot to prevent them from bending over. Bending over while washing feet is another big cause of patients visiting The Back Pain Center. While in the shower, place the foot that needs washing onto the stool while bending the other knee to lower yourself. In this way, you can reach the foot while avoiding as much forward waist bending as possible. Note that any bending that you *must* do should always be performed with abdominals engaged. What does this mean? Imagine you wanted to brace yourself for someone about to punch your stomach – you would tighten up your muscles to protect yourself. By engaging the muscles now, you help lock in the SI joint. That's why, for example, it's a good thing to do if getting in and out of a chair since it helps support the area.

On the other hand, if you are a flexion type patient, depending on your degree of pain, showering while standing can be okay. However, you may require a stool to sit on while washing. If so, you can do some beneficial exercises seated in the shower. Facing away from the showerhead, bend forward and touch the floor like in the seated toe touch described in the previous chapter. You can also cross your ankle over your other knee and lean forward. Then, repeat on the other side. This will help stretch the tendons and ligaments in the hip area. If you've had a hip replacement, do not do this exercise.

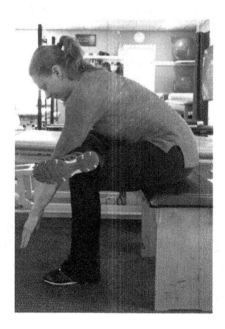

Also, see if you can move your back into a little extension by lifting your chest and leaning backwards *very slightly*.

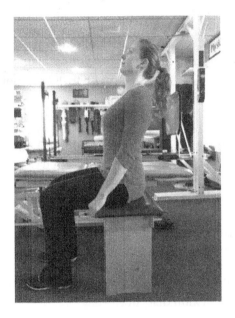

Flexion patients need to regain motion that has been lost, and any opportunity to increase the ability to extend backward should be taken, provided it isn't producing pain. Regaining extension for most flexion patients is a slow process. But be aware: if out of frustration you decide, "Oh, it's just not worth it," and allow yourself to lose some ground, it may not be recoverable.

Walking

Walking is not only our essential method of traveling from one place to another, but can also be great exercise. Whether used for transportation or a workout, it's important to walk with good posture.

For the extension patient – walk tall. Here at **The Back Pain Center**, we say "BBH" a hundred times a day. It stands for breast bone high. Elevating the breast bone upward *but not outward* will almost force you to have good posture. If you're the type to look down at the sidewalk in front of you while walking, then I can assure you that your walking posture is off. Walking is also a good time to incorporate diaphragmatic breathing, as described in chapter 11.

The biggest difference between the flexion patient and the extension patient is that walking is beneficial to the extension patient, while it can be quite an irritation to the flexion patient. They may walk a certain distance and get very tired or achy and have to sit. In fact, walking can act as a good barometer for the progress they are making with their home exercise program. Until they stabilize, if flexion patients are walking and pain becomes problematic, I would then suggest a support to take some of the stress off the spine – a back support, cane, or walker, depending on the severity of the flexion disorder.

Here is some advice that is applicable for all categories of patients with respect to items people carry as they walk. Clearly, it's best not to be encumbered with extra weight or items while walking. Such items can throw off your posture or even balance. For instance, if you are obligated to carry a briefcase, it will obviously place more weight on one side of your body than the other. There aren't any great solutions to this other than to keep it as light as possible and switch sides periodically.

Lifting

If you're at a point in your care where you feel that you are ready to get back into normal daily activities, realize that there are proper and improper ways of lifting.

You significantly increase pressure on the discs if you bend over and lift, rather than just lifting upright. If the object is on the floor, don't bend over to pick it up, but go straight down as if doing a squat. Then, come straight up while keeping your abdominal muscles engaged and tight. Keep your back as vertical as possible, and keep the object as close to your body as you can, with your feet firmly planted and wide apart.

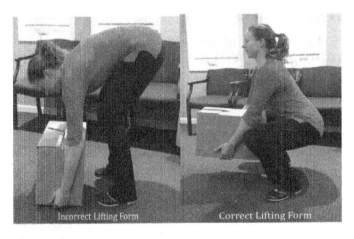

Incorrect Lifting Form   Correct Lifting Form

But before you lift any objects, you really need to have a good idea of how heavy it is. If you're lifting and the object is already up to your knees by the time you realize that it's too heavy, you may have already done much damage. You must assess the weight of an object beforehand and, if need be, put your ego aside and say to yourself, "You know what, I really don't want to lift this. It's too much."

In addition, when lifting and holding weight in your hands, *never* rotate a portion of your body in order to move it. By that I mean, if you have something of weight in your hands that you need to place on a table, don't keep your feet stationary and turn from the waist up – this is an invitation for disaster. You need to *turn your whole body* by moving your feet to point in the direction you wish to face and letting your body follow naturally.

Going To The Bathroom

If you are in an acute state of pain, the actual pressure and strain that you exert to push out a bowel movement can cause the disc to herniate even more. So, if you're in that acute stage, it may benefit you to take a stool softener to make things a little easier and to reduce strain.

Standing At A Workstation Or While Cooking

This can be a killer for the extension type patient whose job requires them to stoop over all day. As discussed in the section on brushing your teeth, try to lean into the tabletop or counter (at a workstation or in the kitchen) and create an arch in the low back area. Moving into this position periodically will reduce the probability of throwing out your back. I also recommend placing a piece of dense foam between your stomach and the tabletop or counter to act as a cushion as you lean. This way, you can lock your legs while maintaining a nice arch in your back, which takes stress off of the back area and will go a long way to keep you from injuring or reinjuring your back.

As for the flexion patient, bending forward with this kind of job or activity isn't generally a problem as their body is adapted to that position. The problem is that the *standing itself* becomes very difficult. For the flexion type patient, finding a relatively high bar stool will help you get through the day. Sit tall on the edge of the stool with feet firmly on the floor; just make sure that you and the stool are stable. In addition, every so often, elevate the chest area, which will introduce motion into the back.

Driving

Getting in and out of a car can be quite a challenge for back pain sufferers. If you have the luxury of choosing which car to drive, choose one that is higher off the ground so you don't have to lower or raise yourself as much to get in and out of the car.

When getting into the car, turn your back to the seat and while holding the door and the body of the car for support, slowly lower yourself into the seat while engaging your abdominal muscles at the same time. Once seated, slowly rotate to face forward, and get your bottom as far back into the chair as possible.

Once seated, the extension patient should use a McKenzie lumbar roll. Also, bring the seat as vertical and forward as possible so that there is as much bend in the knee as possible while still being able to drive safely. When driving, be sure to practice your forward pelvic tilt. Even better, try to synchronize pelvic tilting with diaphragmatic breathing: breathe in when tilting forward, and breathe out when flattening out your back.

Overall, the flexion patient has no trouble with driving. But once again, here is an opportunity to get motion into the spine. In all probability, using a McKenzie lumbar support would irritate the flexion type patient. What *would* be beneficial is trying to lift your breast bone up slowly while your bottom is seated as far back as possible, which will introduce motion into the lumbar area.

The SI patient should follow the same recommendations as for the extension type patient. However, if the pain is located more to one side, you could try doing the seated bike exercise – where one knee is pushed forward while the other is pulled backward, and then the process is reversed. This is great to do if you are a passenger in the car, but please be aware that *if you are driving* and want to attempt this exercise, your safety and that of others around you is paramount. Therefore, if you have any concerns that this exercise could reduce your ability to drive, it should not be done. If that's the case, try contracting your abdominal muscles and do very controlled pelvic rolling forward and back.

For extended drives, regardless of the type of patient you are, use your car's cruise control if you have the opportunity and it would be safe to do so. The subtle position of having one foot slightly forward (constantly on the accelerator) for long periods while driving can be an issue for people with back problems. Using the cruise control allows you to have your foot off the accelerator so your feet can be placed evenly. Additionally, if you are taking a long dive, it's not a bad idea to stop periodically to walk, or even do some of your back exercises! We've had some patients bring along an exercise mat and, while at a rest stop, place it on the grass to do their program.

Shoveling Snow

There is nothing good about shoveling snow, other than filling hospitals with heart attack victims or sending patients to back pain centers. Let me say this loud and clear – shoveling is NOT exercise. Even if you don't have a back problem, if you're out of shape and over 40 years old, pay a kid on the block to do it. If you insist on doing it yourself, then only take light amounts of snow at a time onto the shovel, and bend your knees as much as possible. If you have or have had a history of back problems, particularly if you're an extension type patient, be aware that you are entering very dangerous territory. Wear a lumbar support, in addition to bending at the knees and only shoveling small amounts at a time. Rest frequently and do some extension exercises in between. Using a snow blower would be much safer than shoveling, but be aware that a little forward lean while using the blower can also be enough to set off your back. So again, wear a support belt and stand as tall as possible, letting the blower turn itself by using the gears properly. If turning does require some force on your part, keep your hands as close to your body as possible as you do so.

As it is likely that a flexion patient is older or a senior, just due to age, they should not be shoveling but will do fine with a snow blower. They just need to make sure that they are not pulling or pushing too much to turn the blower around.

Taking Care Of The Lawn

One big difference I have seen between taking care of the lawn and shoveling snow is that there are a good number of patients who actually enjoy doing lawn care, as hard as that is for me to understand. For me to tell them to delegate it to a landscaper generally goes in one ear and out the other. So when using a lawnmower, follow the same principles as with the snow blower. Also, if you need to pull weeds, don't bend over. Get a foam pad from your gardening store and kneel on it instead. Plus, remember the back enjoys motion. Every so often, get on all fours and do some pelvic tilting. While the extension patient should place more emphasis on the arched back with the downward bend, the flexion patient should put more on the camel back with the upward bend.

Jogging

Running is one of those activities where people say, "Doc, I don't care if it's a problem – I love running!" But if you're going to run, you need to be very aware of your posture. Too often, I see people jogging so slowly on the street that I could *walk* faster. I literally want to stop them.

Why? They usually have poor posture and they are just pounding up and down, generally doing more harm than good overall because they are irritating their knees, hips, and low back. Most joggers never fully extend their legs, and as a result, get very tight hamstrings. When I treat joggers, I often find that they've lost all flexibility in their hamstrings.

Another aspect to address is the running surface. A street or sidewalk is a hard, unforgiving surface that is very rough on a body (as is the unevenness of the surface). I have also seen many people develop back problems from running on the side edge of the street next to the sidewalk. Besides being a hard surface, there is a slight slant or bevel in the surface to drain away rainwater. Over time, that alone is enough to cause distortion and change in the low back. The same is true for running on the beach. As picturesque as it looks, the shore has a significant slant to it as well, and could cause the same distortion and subsequent back issues.

If you have the opportunity to do so, I recommend going to a high school track with a composite surface, which is much gentler on the body. Before you start running, walk as part of your warm up – walk quickly until your muscles feel loose. Then stretch your quadriceps (muscles on the front of the thighs) and hamstrings (muscles on the back of the thighs). And when you run – *run*. The faster you run and maintain a steady speed with your chest tall, the better. This posture and pace yields much less trauma on your joints and back.

Most people run for cardiovascular benefit, yet there are studies that question how much running is actually beneficial, and when it becomes detrimental. A heart is a muscle and you *can* overwork it.

I strongly recommend what I call the "kangaroo jog," which means you do a series of 20-second runs in which you are running at a consistent speed. Be clear that this is not a sprint. It's not starting off so fast that you will have slowed down at the end of 20 seconds (which would happen in a 20 second sprint). You want a speed that you can maintain over 20 seconds. Then, at the end of those 20 seconds, check your pulse rate. Does it recover quickly? By the time you walk around the rest of the track to the starting point, it should be back to normal. A healthy heart is one that can recover quickly. If yours does recover fully on the walk back, then do another 20 second burst. If it doesn't recover quickly – you've had enough exercise for the day and you may just want to finish with walking.

As you continue doing this routine, you'll get to a point where your pulse recovers rather quickly. Besides being a great exercise for your body overall, if you run with the proper posture, you'll find that it's also beneficial for your heart.

Please note that before starting this or any exercise, you should always consult your doctor for a realistic appraisal of what you can expect and how aggressively you should approach the exercise.

Shoes

While obviously not an activity, shoes do play a role in every activity we do on our feet, so it is vital to have the proper footwear for good back health. The first question to answer is: do you have any foot abnormalities? Foot pronation (where the heel bone angles inward and the arch tends to be collapsed) or supination (where the body is supported mainly on the anterior, or outside, of the feet) can each interfere with back function.

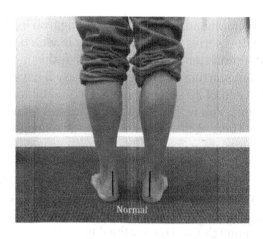

Normal

Foot pronation changes the relationship between the two bones that come up from your ankle to your knee (tibia and fibula), distorting your knee and actually causing a premature arthritis or degeneration of the knee. Fortunately, there are some very simple solutions to a pronated foot with the use of orthotics. When you strike the ground while walking or running, orthotics distribute the weight evenly over the foot, up the leg, and into the hip, thereby reducing any chance that your abnormal foot patterns or your gait will irritate the low back.

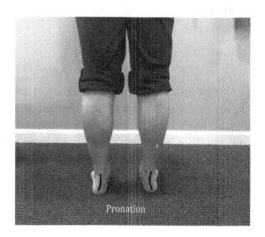

Pronation

Supination is a much more rare foot distortion and should be evaluated by a podiatrist that specializes in this type of disorder.

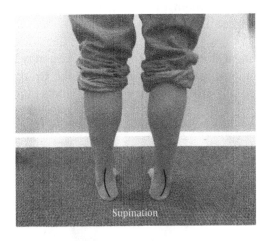
Supination

Other than that, there is no need to see a podiatrist and purchase $300-$500 orthotics. There are effective over-the-counter orthotics in the $50–$65 range, provided they are chosen by a trained podorthist (someone who specializes in proper footwear for patients). They assess how you walk to determine which orthotic would be best for you.

Biking

Biking can be great exercise. However, when biking, you should not sit with your back vertical. You want to lean somewhat forward, with most of your weight on your hands, which is a better posture for your back and places most of the stress on your arms rather than your back. In addition, on the downward motion of your pedaling, your leg should be *almost straight* – just a slight bend. If you're going to bike, it's worth getting measured by someone at the store (ideally someone experienced with bikers and back issues), and even spending a little extra money to get the correct bike.

I also want to point out that most bicycle seats are designed for racing and are not the most comfortable or supportive for your sits bones and back. I have seen ergonomic seats for bikes with splits in them, providing a wider saddle that may provide more comfort for your sit bones.

If you're using a stationary bike at a gym, you may have access to something called a recumbent bike. On this bike, you're essentially sitting down with the pedals in front of you.

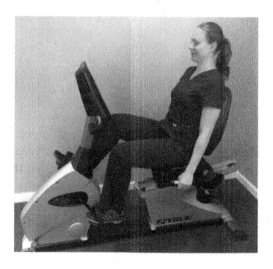

A flexion patient will have no problem using this, but an extension type person should NOT use this type of bike, as it will only aggravate the discs. An SI patient should generally avoid bicycles and opt for walking, elliptical, or treadmill, provided they stand tall. Alternatively, the bicycles used in spinning classes where you lean forward with your weight on your hands would be fine for an extension patient.

However, the problem with many gym exercises classes – especially spin classes – is that you may be next to young men and women who can go two hours at top speed, which may embarrass you to no end! Just realize that *you* need to start out on a gradient. Do it at your own pace, and remember that once you irritate an area, your threshold for reinjuring it drops and it becomes a greater possibility. Depending on your situation, ten minutes of exercise can be great, while more could be detrimental. So when starting out, you are better off starting slowly and building gradually.

Golfing

Golfing is an activity you can do long throughout your lifetime, provided it is done properly and you do exercises supportive of your back. While I cannot claim that it's a great sport for your back, it is one of the few where seniors can maintain some integrity... and where you can get your butt whipped by a 75-year-old.

I have seen golf books and some instructors advise the golfer to maintain an arch in the low back as they swing the golf club. Although this may be good advice for bending forward to brush your teeth or doing the dishes, it is not good advice for the golf swing. Instead, when addressing the ball, you should bend forward and keep your back flat – not arched. Breathe out, tighten your abdominals, and rotate – this way you shouldn't cause yourself problems. Your lumbar spine is actually designed to rotate, and the rotation in golf isn't a problem, *except* if you're arched. The lumbar spine is not designed to rotate in that position, so the golf swing will be significantly more irritating to the joints of the back and the discs if the arch is maintained.

Like with any sport, it's also important to prepare for golfing. Do your stretches and basic exercises. Get to the course early enough to get in some practice swings before you start playing, as a common cause of injury is people starting without warming up.

As you can see throughout this chapter, there are proper or neutral approaches to activities for your back, and others that are harmful. Don't expect that just because you've done a certain activity all your life and have never had a problem that it will always continue to be safe for your back. Heed the advice in this chapter, and seek additional consul from your chiropractor regarding any other activities not mentioned here.

Chapter 19
Sex And Back Pain

Not Tonight, Honey, I Have A *Back*ache

Back pain can interfere with your sex life physically, as well as be an emotionally painful issue for you and your partner, especially if the back issue becomes chronic. Let me state that if you are a back pain sufferer, but sex is not a problem, then feel free to bypass this chapter. I certainly don't want to plant worries where none exist. Many people with back pain are fine, sexually.

On the other hand, for many, back pain can make sex physically difficult and can cause emotional concerns as a result of the inability to care for your partner in ways you did prior to developing back pain. The perceived inability to satisfy one's partner sexually can lead to anger, frustration, apathy, and even depression. This negative impact on what had been a loving relationship is quite common for the patient with chronic, debilitating back pain.

Now, depending on where your sex life was prior to back pain, communication at some level is essential to get things moving forward again. Perhaps not physically back to the level they once were, but definitely to a point where sex is fun and enjoyable again for you and your partner. If your relationship was at all on shaky ground prior to your back pain, then professional help might be considered to help resolve this added dilemma.

The bottom line is that *no communication* can only lead to a greater disconnection. Getting your feelings out and expressing them freely to your partner can go a long way by reconnecting you both and starting the recovery cycle.

Does your partner know how you feel? Are you angry? Do you feel undeserving? Do you feel like you've let your family and your partner down? Are you feeling ashamed? Are you embarrassed or concerned about things getting worse? Has your inability to satisfy your partner made you insecure about your manhood or womanhood? Are you jealous, wondering if your partner is thinking of finding another partner?

Honest communication can only make things better. We have all experienced what it's like to get something off our chest and feel the weight come off our shoulders. Sharing your feelings just might get your sex life going again – and get your back feeling better too. The mind and body are intricately connected. I'm not saying a back problem is just in your mind, but rather, strong negative emotions about it can increase physical tension and stress, therefore exacerbating the problem. Talking is key.

However, your partner or even therapist is not necessarily the only persons with whom you should discuss this issue. If you are comfortable sharing your concerns about sex – and one of those concerns is that having sex may cause more pain or injury – then call your back pain doctor. It can be a chiropractor, physical therapist, or medical doctor specializing in back pain – just make sure they have a high level of expertise regarding back pain. They can help determine what is or is not of genuine concern.

The truth is that when it comes to back disorders, 99 percent of the problems regarding sex are between your ears. Our worries are often much more severe than the actual risks of sex to our backs. With most back problems, sex can still be enjoyable and exciting.

154

Charlie, a 55-year-old male, now on permanent disability following three back surgeries, keeps his wife smiling and has a successful sexual and emotional marriage. Charlie will be the first to share the fact that he is not the man he used to be, sexually. But through communication, acceptance that life changes, and the use of a little imagination and creativity, sex is alive and well in their household.

Unfortunately, the number of patients who come into my office and openly ask about how to deal with back pain and sex is quite small due to the fact that it's an uncomfortable subject. Let me answer some of those questions for you.

Depending on the type of back problem you are dealing with, there are different positions that are safe and will not aggravate your back. If your back problem is related to a sacroiliac joint disorder, disc degeneration, spinal stenosis, or what I classify as a flexion type disorder, then laying on your back with your partner on top should be okay.

On the other hand, if you are dealing with a disc herniation or an extension type disorder, then being on your back might not be the best for you. Being on top and using your arms for support might be more advantageous. Try different side positions too. In most cases, being on your side with the pain side up is helpful.

Doggie style is also fine, provided that the person with a flexion type disorder, disc degeneration, spinal stenosis, or sacroiliac disorder is on the bottom. However, if the back pain sufferer is male and dealing with a disc herniation, then standing, with his partner on all fours on an elevated surface, may be a safe position – that way the male can stand straight without stooping over.

155

Let's say you read this chapter and a described position fits perfectly with your condition and situation, but in trying it out you notice it creates a lot of pain. Even though it is suggested in this book, if the actual experience is hurting, you need to be creative and add your own variations – try lifting one leg a bit or put a pillow under your hips.

The key thing to know is that it's okay to feel a little ache during sex. Don't be so afraid of your back. Some people worry that the wrong move will be the straw that breaks the camel's back (no pun intended), but that break will not happen so easily. You may irritate things and that's okay. One exception to this is if you start to have sex and notice a pain in one of your legs, then you have to stop.

So, experiment. Ultimately, you have to be proactive to stay sexually active. It's up to you to avoid the road of self-pity, guilt, blame, and shame. Realize that things change. Get rid of the hang-ups and realize that none of us are the same as we were 10 or 20 years ago. Also know that there are sexually active seniors well into their 80s having good, enjoyable sex.

If you are depressed about your condition such that sex is literally of no interest – and I appreciate how devastating depression can be – then I understand how it could be upsetting even just reading about the aforementioned positions. In that case, I would again encourage you to seek professional help. Don't give up or give in. Our body's ability to recover can be remarkable. Get the help you need physically *and* emotionally.

Hopefully, recognizing that life isn't always going to be the same as it once was will help with the toughest part when it comes to sex – realizing it's not just a one-person problem. It's only fair to your partner to open up and discuss that things have changed – but that you can both still have fun.

Talk about what positions you want to try and why. He or she probably knows something is going on regardless. If you don't convey to them that some position hurts and you start to retreat, they may misinterpret it as a personal rejection when that's not the case at all.

Sometimes talking about a difficult subject and getting through a tough back experience can have the benefit of bringing two people closer together – even making the relationship better overall once the back pain is resolved. I can say all this with confidence as I have seen it with my own patients.

Chapter 20

There Is Hope

My final hope is that this book can help you find a way out of the trap in which you find yourself. Since the spectrum of patients reading this book will vary from the young athlete who injured his back four weeks ago to the 85-year-old that has been suffering for years, it is challenging to create a book that will address your exact needs.

However, my ultimate goal is to help you navigate through the maze of unlimited advice, thanks largely to the Internet – some good, some bad, and some even dangerous. There are many competent doctors who can help take you to a point of more relief, functionality, and stability.

If after reading this book you feel the need to speak to me personally, I can be reached at The Back Pain Center, where I will try to help steer you in the direction that's right for you. I do want to emphasize that there is nothing like dealing with a patient in person, so first try to use the tools recommended in this book to find a doctor you can trust. I make no promises that I will resolve your problem, but I do promise to give you 100 percent of my attention and to give the best advice I can to help you feel better. You can text our office hotline at (201) 445-1079 for more information.

I thank you for taking the time to read this book, and I pray God be with you on your journey back to better health.

All the best,

Dr. Alfred Gigante